Praise for *Feed Your Soul*

"Finally, a book that takes you past the diets and to-dos, to the heart of the matter of what's going on inside when it come to loving and nourishing your body and feeling good in it. Witty, real, and wise, it's food for the soul that will show you how to approach what you eat and how you eat with self-love, pleasure, and loving truth."

— **Christine Arylo, MBA,** women's leadership adviser and bestselling author of *Choosing ME before WE*

"Using the ancient wisdom of food as medicine, Carly Pollack is on a mission to end the diet dogma once and for all and help us find just the right medicine for our own bodies. I love her lighthearted style as she applies the spiritual principles of awareness, balance, presence, nonjudgment, vibration, and embodiment to having a body you love and a body that loves you. I'm inspired!"

— **Gail Larsen,** teacher and author of *Transformational Speaking: If You Want to Change the World, Tell a Better Story*

"*Feed Your Soul* is clearly the gift of a wise woman who has penetrated the illusions that lead millions to an endless, frustrating relationship with diets. Carly embraces and embodies the first principle of the great alchemists: 'As above, so below.' She invites you into a loving relationship with yourself so food becomes a blessing; when you live your love, your food becomes alive in you as an embodiment of your love, and love is the ultimate harmony. With Carly's guidance and support, you will learn not only to eat for your unique, individual needs but also to love, honor, and respect yourself; and anyone who finds their center becomes a blessing to the world."

— **Paul Chek, HHP,** founder of CHEK Institute

"I love Carly Pollack's new book, *Feed Your Soul.* It is a real, humbling guide to help you unearth the truth about your relationship with food and with your body, as well as the most important relationship you will ever have — the one with yourself."

— **Rebecca Campbell,** author of *Light Is the New Black*

"Carly Pollack's book is a true transformational resource for anyone desiring to improve their health and lose weight for the last time. Carly takes us to the root of our eating woes: the uncontrolled voices in our heads. The tools in this book will set you on a path to food freedom, disease prevention, and a higher quality of life."

— **Alex Carrasco, MD,** founder of Nourish Medicine and author of *Bloom*

"This hilarious book will guide you to achieve success in the most important aspects of your life. A game changer for anyone stuck in old patterns who desperately wants more for themselves."

— **Lauren Fitzgerald, MD,** host of *FITz & Healthy* podcast

feed your soul

NUTRITIONAL WISDOM
TO LOSE WEIGHT PERMANENTLY
AND LIVE FULFILLED

CARLY POLLACK

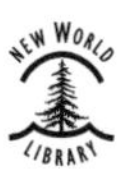

New World Library
Novato, California

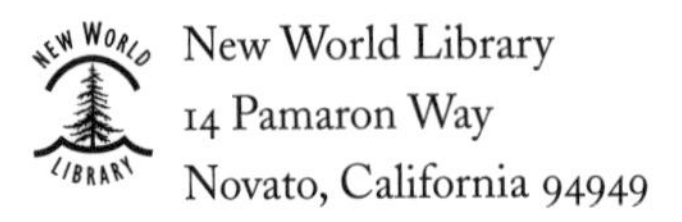

New World Library
14 Pamaron Way
Novato, California 94949

Text design by Tona Pearce Myers

Library of Congress Cataloging-in-Publication Data
Names: Pollack, Carly, date– author.
Title: Feed your soul : nutritional wisdom to lose weight permanently and live fulfilled / Carly Pollack.
Description: Novato, California : New World Library, [2019] | Includes bibliographical references and index.
Identifiers: LCCN 2018047539 (print) | LCCN 2018047905 (ebook) | ISBN 9781608685790 (e-book) | ISBN 9781608685783 (print)
Subjects: LCSH: Weight loss--Popular works. | Weight loss--Psychological aspects--Popular works. | Health behavior. | Nutrition. | Self-care, Health--Popular works.
Classification: LCC RM222.2 (ebook) | LCC RM222.2 .P596 2019 (print) | DDC 613.2/5--dc23
LC record available at https://lccn.loc.gov/2018047539

First printing, February 2019
ISBN 978-1-60868-578-3
Ebook ISBN 978-1-60868-579-0
Printed in the USA on 30% postconsumer-waste recycled paper

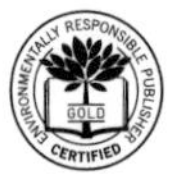

New World Library is proud to be a Gold Certified Environmentally Responsible Publisher. Publisher certification awarded by Green Press Initiative. www.greenpressinitiative.org

10 9 8 7 6 5 4 3 2 1

I dedicate this book to women everywhere
who are working as hard as they can to accept themselves,
while pushing toward something greater.

CONTENTS

Part Three: Find Your True Self

introduction

MAKE IT COUNT

Mental stream #1,235,796: *I am so sick of dieting. There has got to be a more productive way to use my mental energy. I should be curing cancer, fighting for women's rights, or helping starving children in Africa. I bet if I went to Africa I would totally lose weight. Hillary Clinton has a spare tire, but does she obsess over it? No! She's thinking about way more important things than whether or not this morning's treadmill purgatory canceled out last night's pizza binge from hell. I bet Maya Angelou never ate a muffin and then shit-talked herself. Is there ever going to be a time when I don't have to think about this? Stop the insanity, Carly!*

Shit. I pressed snooze one too many times, and now I'm late. The thought of getting out of my warm bed and facing the day ties my stomach into a knot, but my mind is already racing so I figure I might as well get moving. I walk into the bathroom and head right for the scale. I hold my breath, knowing it's not going to be kind after last night's debacle with an entire box of Newman's Own chocolate mint cookies. Here we go. I step onto the scale with one eye squeezed shut, only 50 percent committing to looking at the dreaded number. Yep, there it is. That stupid package of "healthy" cookies has magically already worked its way onto my thighs, and the scale is confirming that I'm a worthless piece of turd with no self-control.

Now that I know my wish of waking up looking like Jessica Alba has once again not come true, I head into the closet for my second shaming of the day, my jeans. I know at this scale weight that the only pair I can choose are my black, elastic, and oh-so-forgiving jeans. My eyes dart over to that evil pair of gray skinny jeans that I bought that one day when I was feeling particularly svelte. I make sure to feel that sting of regret from last night's snack as I grab my black jeans and give up hope that today will be the day that getting dressed is actually enjoyable.

Robotically putting on my makeup, I am anything but present as the voice in my head is going a million miles an hour. I'm planning out my gym schedule for the week, promising my body redemption by Friday. It's Monday, which means I'm back on my diet of protein and vegetables. Carbs are the enemy during the week, but on the weekend I am my own worst enemy. As mental food prison and work anxiety kick into high gear, I'm counting the hours until I can come home, take off my bra, and watch TV with my cat.

This routine used to go on week after week, over and over again, like a show on repeat. My routine: the most inconsistent yet consistent pattern. During the week I exercised and counted out my almonds for my snack, constantly stressing about work and life. On the weekends I broke loose and let go with reckless abandonment. I ate whatever I wanted and avoided any and all responsibility by smoking pot all day long to shut out the little voices in my head. Of course, the dreaded bathroom scale echoed my behavior loud and clear. Throughout the year, I would gain and lose the same ten pounds every month. This cycle left me feeling depleted, annoyed, and guilty.

One day I had an epiphany. Not only was what I was doing not working (that was pretty obvious), but I wasn't happy. I thought I should lose weight to be happy, and for the first time I realized that perhaps I had it completely wrong. Maybe I needed to work on getting happy so that I could finally lose the weight. Maybe there was a lesson I needed to learn, and my weight was a way of telling me I hadn't learned it yet.

This book is about so much more than just what you put into your mouth. In fact, very little of your path to success has anything to do with food. I know, it's hard to believe, but it's true. In fact, I will clear up nutrition for you in about ten minutes, because it really is that simple. The real work will be done inside you, not on your plate. It will be done by looking at your path to health and happiness as something with deeper meaning. It will become a spiritual path, a path to better understand yourself and your place in the Universe.

I am the queen of credentials. I have a bachelor's degree in nutrition and a master's degree in holistic nutrition, I am a certified clinical nutritionist and health and lifestyle coach, and I have specialized study in women's nutrition (I know it's hard to imagine, but I swear I'm still funny at parties). Even with eighteen years of study in the field of nutrition and holistic health, it is my personal experience with my weight and body image struggles that makes me an expert on permanent change.

Through my discovery of what it truly takes to lose weight, ditch the anxiety, and finally live a life in which I feel present, healthy, and happy, I was able to make permanent changes in my body — which were the least of my transformation. If this is something you want to achieve, to become the healthiest and happiest version of you, then get ready for a good brainwashing (because dirty brains need washing).

Before you dive into this book, I want you to set an intention. An intention is a plan that you create before you jump into action. It has been said that "what we believe, we become," and therefore our intentions manifest into our reality. Typically, when I start reading a new book, my unconscious thought process is, "Okay, what's in it for me?" So now I'll ask you, what's in it for you? What do you want to feel, be, or do as a result of learning how to love yourself and care for yourself so that you can make permanent changes in your life and health?

Take a moment and relax into your body. Think about why you picked up this book in the first place. What drew you to it, and why do you want to devote your time to it? Now, create an intention for what you want to receive from these teachings. Each time you pick up this book, give yourself a moment to close your eyes and visualize the intention you will create right here and now. Picture yourself feeling free from the never-ending cycle of dieting. Imagine yourself feeling happy, healthy, and light.

Set a standard for how you will devour this book. Commit to reading every day, even for just a few minutes, for immersion is the best way to create change. Commit to doing the journal entries and exercises. Tell yourself now that you are 100 percent committed to squeezing out every ounce of goodness from this freedom guide.

But first let's have a serious talk about the 5 percent. If you have an exercise routine, you've probably heard that the last few reps are where the change happens. If your workout is forty-five minutes long, minute forty is where the body starts to morph. The hard part is that at this point in the workout, we are exhausted, our form is wavering, and we tell ourselves it's okay to half-ass it because we are almost done. We finish the workout, checking it off a list of to-do's for the day, yet we don't feel like our bodies ever change in any noticeable way. It's that last 5 percent that gets us.

This book also comes with a 5 percent: the "Make It Stick" sections at the end of each chapter, which make the difference between simply reading this book and using it to change who you believe you are and what you are capable of. You must take *massive action* if you want to create change deep within your nervous system. Commit right now to doing that final 5 percent, because you've already done most of the hard work, and you deserve to make it last. Make sure you have a notebook (digital or analog) on hand, and commit to finishing every assignment!

Let's dive in.

PART ONE

retrain the brain

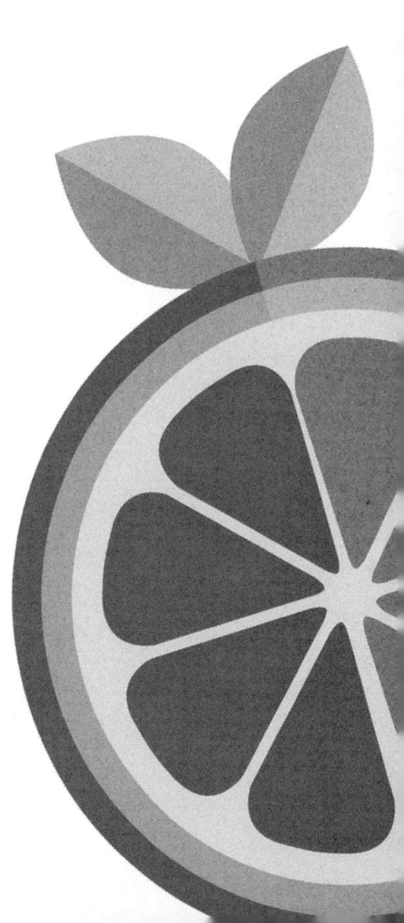

chapter 1

IT'S ALL IN YOUR HEAD

You don't have to believe everything you think.
— My first meditation teacher

The mind is an excellent servant,
but it is a terrible master.
— Robin Sharma

I think it's safe to say that, like most people, you are struggling or have struggled with some pressing issue. You want to improve your career, your relationships, your financial status, or your health. You're worried that you are not good enough, that you could fail, or that bad things will happen. Or maybe you have so much amazing abundance in your life that you are positively scared shitless that it's all going to blow up in your face one day soon.

The second that something wonderful happens in our lives, that little voice inside our head finds a way to allow fear to rain on the parade. I remember wanting a relationship so much, and then the moment I fell in love, I started to have irrational fears about something tragic happening to my partner. Or the time I finally got the job I had worked so freaking hard for and all I could think was, "I won't do a good enough job to make a positive first impression." Do you remember worrying about whether you were going to make friends in college, then making so many friends that you stressed about balancing your social life with your schoolwork? If you don't learn how to control the voice inside your head, this stress-inducing mental prison will only grow more confining over time.

One thing I can guarantee is that the narrative in your head, that incessant stream of chatter, is responsible for all your unrest. Regardless of your specific desires, I know it's peace of mind that you want, because the end goal of all end goals is to be happy! Anytime you want to manifest something in your life, you are being driven by the belief that in having it you will experience happiness.

The problem is that our culture has given us a backward message. It's taught us we must *achieve* to be happy. Have more, do more, become more, so that you can stress less. When Biggie Smalls says, "Mo' money, mo' problems," I interpret that as meaning "achievement without an inner spiritual practice causes nothing but worry." Yes, the Notorious B.I.G. was a hippie sage underneath all those gold chains.

Have you ever thought about why you want to look great in a bathing suit? It's not because you think it will help you live longer. It's because you think that in looking great, you will become more accepted and desired, and that will make you happy. There is absolutely no shame in that belief, and I am here to help you make that sexy beach photo happen! I simply want you to step back and realize that everything you desire right now really comes down to your desire to be happy and at peace.

Side note: There have been times in my life when I was skinny but terribly unhappy (you know that postbreakup, can't-eat, life-is-over kind of skinny), so I know with certainty that deep in our emotional core, the two states are not intrinsically linked.

The Formula That Changed It All

There's a point in the process of dieting, usually close to the beginning, when we experience hopeful euphoria. The diet is working for us, we feel great, and we feel like we've finally got it. It's the point at which we think about our past behaviors and exclaim that we are never going back to that old way of eating again! We are essentially high on the diet, and we want to climb a mountain and scream from the top, "I'm cured!" A few weeks later, we leave our favorite Thai restaurant feeling disgusted (and yet somewhat impressed) with how much pad thai we were able to shove down our gullets. We think back to our mountaintop moment and wonder why and how we have fallen so far from grace. Does restricting our food intake release some special endorphins that make us appear more confident than we really are? If we were truly that happy about all the positive eating changes, then why did we go back to our old patterns?

Because I have visited the mountaintop a time or two (or ten), I have the answer to why we fall so hard from grace and directly into a bag of chips. It is also the key to understanding why diets don't work. Consider this formula:

Thoughts ⟶ Emotions ⟶ Behaviors ⟶ Reward or consequence

Diets don't work because they focus on behavior modification and nothing more. Eat this, don't eat that; and if you eat that, you break the rules of the diet, and that makes you lazy, inadequate, weak, unlovable, and [insert insult] here. If we are brave and vulnerable enough to look more deeply at what truly needs to be healed, we will have success eliminating our negative behaviors at their root. It is our minds that drive the eating bus. In fact, *our thoughts drive every emotion we feel, and how we feel will dictate how we act.* Unless we change the original thought/story, we will re-create the same painful pattern, a nightmarish diet-induced *Groundhog Day.*

For years I went on and off diets, some sane, some downright insane (hello, prepackaged meals and freeze-dried snacks; I want a refund). I went through long periods of reckless abandonment, also known as eating everything I craved until all my clothes stopped fitting. When anything with an elastic waistband became my preferred pants for every outing, I would prepare for my next big diet adventure. Eventually I stopped going for extended periods of time in eating denial. I evolved to binging and restricting all within a week's time.

Monday was always redemption day for me. A fresh start and a new opportunity to finally stop abusing myself with food. I would plan my gym workouts, make my grilled chicken and vegetables, and promise myself that this week would be the start of something permanent. The thought of finally feeling good in my body evoked hopefulness and desire, which changed my eating behavior during the week. But by the end of the week, I was tired, stressed, and ready to break free from the almond-counting food prison of the past five days. It was a subtle shift, but my thoughts changed from "I want to feel good in my body" to "It's the weekend, and I deserve comfort and rewards for all my hard work." That subtle shift in thought created new emotions, which drove unhealthy weekend behaviors time after time. I was the epitome of the weekday warrior and the weekend partier. No diet could save me. If I wanted to make any real, permanent change, I had to look internally to examine the underlying thoughts that were consuming my brain. Once I started using my formula to get to the real root of the issue, true and permanent change emerged.

Your thoughts are most likely subconscious; they ride underneath the surface, and you may not even notice they are there. If you heighten your awareness and start questioning your behaviors with this formula as your guide, you will start to notice that exact moment when your emotional thinking about food changes.

The practice of paying attention to your thoughts can be hard at first, especially if you have been listening to the voice in your head your entire life (and believing every word it says). The easiest way to heighten your awareness is to simply ask yourself throughout the day, "What am I thinking?" If you are a person who can connect more easily with your feelings than your thoughts, identify your emotions and work backward. If you ask yourself, "What am I feeling?" and the answer is, "Stressed and exhausted," then you can take it a step further and ask, "What story am I telling myself right now that is creating this stress?" This is you working your way through the meat of my formula. For the first time, your focus is on what really needs healing and *not* on your plate. By the time you question your eating behaviors, you are too far down the rabbit hole to make any permanent change. (Just a heads-up: Once you start paying attention to your thoughts, you are going to realize that your mind is absolutely insane. You will need to learn how to distinguish between what's real and what's pure crazy, but I'll help you navigate those shark-infested waters.)

To create the life and body you want, you must do so from a place of peace, gratitude, and happiness. You can't fake it. If you're going to achieve deep and fulfilling success, love, and abundance, you have to separate your mind (thoughts) from your heart and soul (your higher self). Only then will you create peaceful behaviors around food.

Strengthen the Higher Self

Before you can regain control of your thoughts, beliefs, and emotional state, you must first take a closer look at your internal guidance system. Two different voices are guiding you, and although they both *sound* like you, one is a much pushier, more obnoxious version and therefore steals most of your attention. This loud voice comes from your monkey mind, which I simply call the "mind" and many spiritual teachers call the "ego."

The mind developed as a way to protect us; it was a means of survival. It helped us avoid danger and kept us alive by continually warning us of what could go wrong. As we have evolved as a species, the mind, sadly, has not. Think of it as an outdated computer that drives you crazy more than it helps you get things done. Now, I'm not saying the mind doesn't step up in life-or-death situations. I'm talking about the other 99.999 percent of the time here.

The mind creates chaos through fear, judgment, comparison, and negativity. Its favorite diatribe is the one that convinces us of scarcity. We aren't pretty, skinny, or rich enough. There isn't enough time in the day, there aren't enough good people in the world, and we don't have enough willpower to make things happen. Whatever the heck it is, there just isn't enough of it!

The mind's second favorite story is that something is happening or has happened to us that "shouldn't be" happening (or "shouldn't have" happened). It convinces us that we aren't supposed to have problems — and when we do, the mind creates massive suffering. The mind is excellent at dress-rehearsing a worst-case scenario. It finds a way to judge and blame as much as possible. If you aren't judging someone else, then you are judging yourself. This constant uninvited commentary is the background of your every waking moment. From the minute you open your eyes to the moment your head hits the pillow, your mind does not shut up. Yeah, mind, I'm calling you out big-time, and I'm telling you to take a backseat; and PS, nobody likes you.

Luckily, there is a second guiding voice, and this one comes from your heart and soul, otherwise referred to as your intuition, true self, or inner wisdom. I like to call this voice my "higher self" because it triggers me to think about what I would say to myself if I were holding myself in the highest regard. Find a name for this place of wisdom that feels good to you, and begin to call on this voice to take the upper hand. Your higher self comes through in a whisper, a gentle guidance. It is always kind, compassionate, and loving. This voice lives only in the present moment, and it is available to us anytime we can quiet the mind enough to hear it. From this place, we are never arguing with "what is" because we are living in the moment, making new decisions as they arise.

Close your eyes right now (well, after you read these instructions) and place your right hand on your belly and your left hand over your heart. Take three slow, deep breaths. Now ask yourself gently, "What does my higher self have to say about this issue?" If you don't hear anything right away, simply say, "I'm willing to slow down my mind and make room for my highest wisdom to come through."

Because your mind has taken center stage for most of your life, it may take some practice to get your higher self to begin speaking up. Next time you are in a place of mental anguish, prompt yourself with the following questions:

- What would I tell my best friend in this situation? What would be my sage advice?
- Could this mean something different? What if the opposite of what I'm thinking is true?
- What would love do? What would love say?
- What do I think my future self (twenty years from now) would tell me about this problem or situation?

Listening to your higher self is the first step to taking back control from the mind. Witnessing your thoughts without giving in to them, while stepping back and deciding what you *choose* to think, is one of the most powerful tools you have for living a joyful life. If you control your mind, you control your plate. If you control your plate, you take back control of your body and your health.

I grew up on Staten Island. It took only twenty-five minutes to get over the bridge into Manhattan. I was (and still am) obsessed with Broadway, so my parents would take my sister and me into the city to see all the shows, eat at all the new restaurants, and check out the museums. One of my favorite things to do was to sit in a restaurant, facing the window, and people-watch. I would see a melting pot of fashion, attitude, and ethnicity. I was in awe of everyone's individuality.

I would make up stories about the people walking by. One was a famous fashion photographer on his way to a shoot. The other was a Wall Street finançier meeting a client for lunch. The hippie chick was a singer/songwriter trying to get her big break in the city. I would wonder what these people were thinking. Imagine, in a busy city like New York, if everyone said out loud what they were thinking. Can you picture the herds of people walking down the street, vocalizing the thousands of thoughts that run through their heads? As different as everyone looks, I bet their thoughts would be disappointingly ordinary. The specific stories would alter slightly based on the person, but there would be a standard pattern of thinking. We would hear fear, judgment, comparison, and worst-case-scenario thinking. We would hear stories told from only one perspective in a random and unnecessary monologue. We would notice that there wasn't much space in between these rapid-fire thoughts, and that they were mostly negative. We would witness the similarities of the mind. Think about your incessant stream of thoughts when you are in the car, the shower, at work. If you spoke these thoughts aloud, you could quite possibly be diagnosed as insane!

Improve Your Food Karma

Remember the time when you were in full premenstrual swing and you called your girlfriend to meet at your favorite restaurant for a salad? No, you don't, because that never happened. I bet you do remember sitting on the couch watching a rom-com from the '80s and eating an entire bag of chips, followed by half a jar of peanut butter while wondering how Julia Roberts stayed so damn skinny. In fact, I'd like you to think back to all the times you felt miserable, sad, angry, or depressed. What kind of food did you crave? My guess is that it wasn't a salad or a green juice.

The vibrational law of attraction applies to everything in life, and eating is no exception. I call it "food karma." The law of karma is "like attracts like." The law of attraction is that what you put out (thoughts, words, actions) will come right back to you. Ponder that for a moment. Simply put, *when you feel bad, you are going to crave foods that, after eating them, will make you feel even worse.* Americans create a lot of confusion by calling certain foods "comfort foods." They are supposed to ease our uncomfortable emotional state. I'd like to find someone who feels comfortable after eating fried chicken and mashed potatoes. "I just got fired, but this fried chicken is so good. Now I know that next great job is right around the corner." I don't know about you, but I can't wait to go for a five-mile run right after eating some chicken pot pie. What we think is comforting is just numbing, and afterward, we feel just as uncomfortable as we did before we ate the pot pie, except what was once just emotional discomfort has now turned into physical discomfort (and probable weight gain, which is translated into long-term emotional and physical discomfort) as well. When I have one problem, I like to solve that one problem instead of doing/eating something that creates another problem. What about you? If you had a choice between having one problem or two, what would you choose?

Every thought we think emits a vibration. There is no neutral here; every thought you have could be classified as putting out either a positive, uplifting, loving energy or a negative, Debbie Downer, fear-based energy. We could rate each emotion on a scale, with love, gratitude, and empowerment being at the top and fear, grief, hopelessness, and stress being at the very bottom. If you want to be a vibrational match to healthy foods that make you feel and look fantastic, you need to work your way up the emotional scale by shifting your story.

Failure Feels Like French Fries

It took me three years to be eligible to sit for my certified clinical nutritionist exam. It required one year of study post–master's degree, which I had to complete in little spurts while I was growing my private practice. Having this certification meant everything to me. Everyone in my field whom I looked up to had these initials after their name; plus it would allow me to order lab work and help my clients find more answers to their health woes. Studying for this mind-numbing test was like studying for the SAT and GRE combined.

Normally I am overly confident when it comes to being a student. I'm the girl at the front of a class, handing in her paper early while being intensely hated by all the students suffering from chronic procrastination and a hangover. But this test had me nervous. I was a walking cue card by the week of the exam. I remember sitting in front of the computer, praying to God, Lord Ganesh, the angels, and my dead grandparents to help me pass this test. Three hours, four bathroom breaks, long periods of panic, and brief moments of confidence later, I found myself staring at a screen that had nothing on it except a button that said "Submit test to see score." I needed a score of 75 to pass. I took a deep breath, closed my eyes, and hit the mouse clicker for the final time.

I opened my eyes to see this on the screen: "You received a 74/100. You did not pass this test. Please call your administrator to reschedule this test for a later date. Thank you." All the saliva in my mouth spontaneously evaporated, and I swallowed what felt like a sheet of sandpaper. My stomach started turning, and I sat there stunned for what felt like ten minutes (but was probably closer to thirty seconds). I scooted my chair back and got up slowly as tears filled my eyes. The first overwhelming emotion I felt was shame.

Everyone close to me knew I was taking this test. What was I going to say to my employees, who were waiting to celebrate this milestone with me? I was their mentor, and now I have to go back and tell them that I failed by one measly point? I got into my car and started ugly crying. With snot running down my face, I clutched the steering wheel, rocked back and forth, and wept, while praying that no one passing my car would notice. After a few minutes of *Jerry Springer Show*–quality behavior, I calmed down and decided I had two choices.

I could open Google Maps and find the closest hole to crawl into, or I could go home and find "comfort."

My mother was waiting for me as I walked in the door. She took one look at my face and said, "Okay...okay. Let's go eat somewhere. I'll take you anywhere you want to go. What do you want to eat?" All the fried, sugary, most calorie-dense foods scrolled through my mind. If I was going to give myself a free pass to feel bad, I'd better choose something really worth it. I mean, if I'm in hell already, why not feed the flames, right? Perhaps it was my emotional breakdown that had left me unable to bullshit myself, but that moment with my mom slapped me into clarity. I had been using food my entire life to alter my emotional state because I didn't have the tools to alter it myself. All those past diets and exercise regimes were no match for the emotional codependency I had created with food.

The foods we crave are entirely dependent on our emotional state, which you now know is completely reliant on our thought process. *No matter how logical a diet seems, it ultimately fails to heal our food issues at the root.* According to the law of attraction, changing our behavior with food could never work in the long term because it's our negative emotions that block us from maintaining the vibrational match to healthy, high-vibration foods. When you feel bad, you are not a vibrational match for healthy foods that make you feel good. If you feel bad and by some miracle you are eating well despite yourself, then be careful, because you are using pure willpower, and that, my friend, is quite a limited resource!

Because I would never leave you hanging, I'll tell you the ending to this test-taking melodrama. Since I ain't no quitter, I called the certification board and demanded that they review my test, since I felt there were at least a few questions that had more than one right answer. They agreed and wound up passing me by two points. Needless to say, the head of the board had an Edible Arrangement coming to her. I sprung for the chocolate-dipped fruit, because I like to keep it classy.

Willpower vs. Discipline

My only goal for my first Mexican getaway with my (then) boyfriend was to look outstanding in a bathing suit. Naturally, that meant going on some strict crash diet weeks beforehand and working out as if I was training for the Olympics. For three weeks, whenever I wasn't on dates with Jordan, I was on dates with the treadmill. On previous vacations, I had made the mistake of getting in shape for the trip, and then as soon as I arrived at my destination I would eat junk that bloated me to high heaven for the rest of the vacay. That bloat wasn't going to get me down this time. Hell, no! I was going to keep it together during the trip and stick to the food plan. If you had asked me why I wanted to look so perfect, I couldn't have given you an answer that was rooted in anything substantial, certainly not anything having to do with self-love. I was doing it out of fear. I wanted to look good in photos so that when I posted them, other people would validate me. I wanted my partner to validate me through his attraction to me. I believed the story that my appearance was directly related to my worth.

We all want so badly to feel worthy, to feel *enough*. Instead of driving ourselves crazy trying to prove our worthiness, why don't we just decide we are enough, just because we get up every day and try to be better versions of ourselves?! End of story. From here on out, that is going to be our only requirement of worthiness, to wake up with a desire to grow as a human being. I'm here to tell you that not only are you enough, but that sometimes you are too damn much.

If we are to free ourselves from the fear-based, ill-fated practice of willpower, we need to shift emotions and play this game from a different angle. *The opposite of fear is love.* Everything rooted in fear is an illusion (much more on this later, so sit tight). Everything rooted in love is real. Wanting to look good from a place of love means wanting your physical body to reflect how much you genuinely love and care about yourself. Wanting to look great in a bikini on a beach vacation is fantastic, as long as this desire comes from the place of wanting to feel good digestively, and energetically, so that you can be more conscious to the present moment and the adventure unfolding before you. It comes down to changing your story about why you want the things you want. At the root, your desire always needs to come from a place of wanting to be able to enjoy more of life's pleasures. This raises your vibrational frequency to an energetic state that attracts more positive foods and fulfilling experiences.

For the first few days of vacation, I kept it together by using willpower. Willpower comes from the energy of fear. It creates thoughts like "I shouldn't eat this. I want this, but I can't have it." Even if you prevail, it creates a feeling of lack, aka not-enoughness. Willpower gets weaker the more we use it, which is why we always wind up eating doughnuts and skipping our workout later in the day. What do you expect? You've used willpower all day long. You smiled at your wretched coworker, you wrote a nice email to the client who just gave you attitude, you did an hour of yoga while smelling the girl next to you who makes her own deodorant but smells like she forgot to wear it, and you sat through forty-five minutes of traffic without flipping anyone off. Your willpower is toast. How could you *not* eat your entire pantry as if you were expecting Armageddon? You've got nothing left holding you back from those two-week-old crackers.

After a few days of vacation, I burned through all my willpower. I was done. What followed were corn chips at lunch and dinner, plus that plate of morning pastries that I had been eyeing all week. By the end of the vacation, I felt the way I always did: bloated, guilty, constipated, and promising myself a cleanse upon my return. And so the diet struggle continued.

If the opposite of fear is love, then *the opposite of willpower is discipline.* Discipline comes from a place of love. Discipline sounds like this: "I love the way that food tastes, but I love myself more." Using discipline feels great; you feel empowered and crystal clear about what you truly want. You are unwilling to give up what you want most for what your mind is saying you want right now. Conversely, when you are using willpower alone, you are pissed off at yourself, even after you have made the right choice. You feel imprisoned by food and indebted to some old behavior. Three days later you eat something even worse than the food you avoided, just to spite yourself.

Since all our food issues begin in our head, we must realize that food prison is a state of mind. When we go on diets, we start eating healthfully, but all the old stories keep us stuck. We might be following the rules, but it's because we have to, not because we want to. We want the fries, but we order the salad. Great! Now we are in lettuce jail. We feel tremendous scarcity around food, and it makes us feel crazy.

As we begin to uncover our negative thoughts and shift them, we realize that boundaries around food create body freedom, not food prison. We start eating in a way that makes us feel free on a much deeper level than "free to eat whatever we want." We begin to feel free in our bodies and our experiences. We start to find deeper meaning and joy that wasn't available to us when we were stuck in the mental roller coaster of food and body obsession. This foundational mental shift is the only thing that can truly set us free.

I know this is much easier said than done, but the good news is that you need only one tool to begin the practice of changing your thoughts: awareness. As discussed earlier, start checking in with yourself throughout the day by asking a straightforward question: "What am I thinking?" If you are thinking something negative, you know that is foreshadowing for negative behavior. If you are thinking something that brings up negative emotion, well, you are about to eat something terrible, girlfriend! If you are nervous about not being able to increase your awareness around your thoughts, emotions, and behaviors, just take a deep breath, and say to yourself, "I trust myself to be aware with ease," and read on.

Skimmer's Delight

- ✓ Thoughts → Emotions → Behaviors → Reward or consequence
- ✓ You receive guidance from two places: the mind and your higher self.
- ✓ You must begin the practice of listening to your higher self to drive different and more positive behavioral outcomes.
- ✓ Every emotion you have puts out a vibration. Negative emotional states create a vibrational match to processed, low-quality foods.
- ✓ When you feel bad, change your thoughts to improve your emotional state. You will naturally start craving healthier foods.
- ✓ Your goal is to love foods that love you back. This may look like a strict diet from an outsider's view, but if you do the mental work and come from a place of discipline (love), you will experience food freedom.

Make It Stick

1. Identify one personal story that fits the ego's favorite two complaints: something is happening (or has happened) that shouldn't be, and feeling as if there's never enough time or enough money or that you never feel good enough. What would your higher self say? How does this change the way you feel and ultimately how you act?
2. Journal about one of your negative food behaviors. What story, and emotion, drives this behavior? Rewrite the story.
3. Set a twice-daily alarm on your phone that says, "What am I thinking?" Take the time to replay some of the stories that you feel will cause a regretful behavior. Rewrite that story from the place of your higher self.

chapter 2

DON'T GIVE UP WHAT YOU WANT MOST FOR WHAT YOU WANT RIGHT NOW

The primary cause of unhappiness is never the situation but your thoughts about it. Be aware of the thoughts you are thinking. Separate them from the situation, which is always neutral. It is as it is.
— **Eckhart Tolle**

When we change the way we look at things, the things we look at change.
— **Wayne Dyer**

Screw it. I had a hard week. I'm eating this, and I don't care.... Whatever — I'm staying up for another episode, even though I'm supposed to wake up early to make that 7 AM *yoga class. I don't care.... I don't care what I wrote in my journal about how to comfort myself without food. I'm PMSing, so bring on the fries.*

We lie to ourselves with embarrassing regularity. I used to lie to myself all the damn time (I still do; I just know how to catch myself now). I think the lie I told myself most often in the moment was that I "didn't care." It wasn't until I started the practice of separating fact from story that I realized this lie was at the root of all my food self-sabotage.

One day, after I had so coolly told myself that I didn't care, my sassy higher self finally spoke up and said, "Stop lying to yourself. Not only do you care, but you care more about this than anything else!"

Fact or Fiction?

Our negative thoughts are very often illusions falsely presented to us as absolute truths. You've been there many times before, thinking you were so sure about a situation or person (or where you left your keys), only to be utterly humbled in your wrongness. At that moment you sat back and thought, "Hmm, I was so sure that…" Only you weren't. You know why? The mind doesn't always tell us the right story. Most of the time we have limited data to begin with, which causes us to weave our hallucination into the black spaces where we have no facts. I am most impressed with my mind when I unknowingly make up an entire story from one single fact.

Single fact: I texted someone, and she has not yet responded.

My story: She never texts me back; it's so rude. She probably looked at her phone, read the text, and didn't even feel like she needed to respond. She is so selfish. If I text her because I need her to do something for me, I never hear back. If she needs something from me, well, then all of a sudden she is readily available…

Then that person texts me back apologizing for not responding sooner because she had a family emergency, and I feel like a piece of crap. If you don't realize that your mind is conjuring up stories like this at least once a day, then that's just another story keeping you from the truth! These stories create massive emotional suffering, which you now know will translate into some poor eating behavior if you don't know how to spot these stories and turn them around while they are still thoughts.

There is a fundamental difference between fact and story. A fact is something that is true for everyone. A story is something you think is true for you based on your perceived reality and belief system. Not all stories are wrong. In fact, I don't want you to live your life only listening to facts: how boring! Instead, I want you to tell yourself positive stories about what you are capable of. I want you to be Positive Pollyanna, skipping around telling yourself stories of empowerment and overall badassery. To live that way, we need to knock out all the Debbie Downer stories that aren't true and are blocking us from living our best lives. To change at the thought level, we need to examine and neutralize the stories we tell ourselves.

Perhaps you look in the mirror and think to yourself, "I'm so fat, I look disgusting." Realize that for that statement to be a fact, for you to fully believe that it is the truth, everyone would need to agree that you are fat and look disgusting. You might be thinking that it's impossible to get everyone on this planet to agree that this is the case, and you would be right. That nasty thought is not a fact; it's a story, and thank goodness for that because a thought that mean and disempowering can and should be changed.

There are three levels of thought, each level more ingrained into your nervous system. The first and most basic level of thought is what I call a "passing thought." You get on an airplane and sit down, and as you watch people walking down the aisle to their seats, your mind presents some passing thoughts. "What if this plane crashed and these people are the last people I ever see? If the plane went down, would I grab my purse? There's a mirror in there; I bet I could use it to catch the attention of the rescue helicopter. Okay, stop being ridiculous, the plane will be fine. Let's see what free movies they're showing on this little screen here." These thoughts don't carry much weight; they pass through you without causing too much of an emotional reaction. You need to start cataloging your passing thoughts as positive or negative. The negative ones you let pass through you, and the positive ones you hold on to and repeat over and over again until they become beliefs.

David is a client of mine who came in weighing 296 pounds. In just a few months he lost fifty pounds. After that, he started plateauing. I asked him why he thought his weight loss had stalled, and he responded, "Well, now is when it's supposed to be hard. I know the last fifteen pounds are going to come off painfully and slowly." I asked him why he thought that and he said, "I dunno, I've seen people around me who have lost the weight, and they always struggle around this point in their journey." I'll call this story the "dreaded last few pounds" story. We have all heard that the last few pounds of weight loss are really stubborn, but have we ever questioned why this story exists? Is it that the body knows this is the last weight to go and purposefully makes it harder to lose, or is it that the dedication required to get in peak condition is not something most people are willing to commit to? Is the weight stubborn to come off, or is it hard to get in the right mental state? The mind loves to confuse correlation with causation.

This level of thought is a *belief.* Beliefs are created through stories (which are a string of thoughts) that have been validated through experience, either yours or someone else's. This level of thought is a little stickier, since the mind has an experience that proves it to be "true." Are theories true sometimes? Yes, but the false-versus-true-theories ratio is way off, and not in our favor. Tip: It's useful to use the word *theory* when talking about your beliefs. It helps you realize that what you are thinking may not be true. If you are looking in the mirror while bathing suit shopping, you could say, "It's my theory that I don't look good in these bathing suits" instead of "I am a fat cow, and it should be illegal for me to wear this in public." See how the word immediately triggers you to realize that your belief is just a theory and not a fact? Once David was able to make this connection, he pushed through his barriers and lost the rest of the weight, a few months after our last meeting. He now participates in torturously long adventure races and carries backpacks, that combined with his body, still weigh less than his starting weight!

The way I lost weight in the past was to go on a strict no-sugar diet for a period of time. I would eat nothing but protein and vegetables with healthy oils, no bread, no pasta, no processed anything. While on paper this is an exceptionally healthy diet, it can drive you a little nuts. I would lose weight and eventually want to eat everything in sight. It never worked long-term, but because it's how I lost weight in the past, anytime I felt like I wanted to drop some pounds, my mind would tell me to follow my old diet theory. The mind is very simple in that way. "Carly wants to lose weight; she does the diet; she loses weight." That theory is now an absolute, a belief that now becomes my reality. It doesn't take into account that I couldn't keep the weight off; it's simply a pattern my mind has created with the limitation that this is the only way to lose because it's worked (temporarily) before.

The best way to uncover your beliefs is to write down "Thoughts I Think about __________" and insert your beliefs into the blank. For example, let's say I write "Thoughts I Think about My Body" and then make a list and allow the judgment, ranting, and random descriptions to flow onto the paper. If one of my thoughts is that my body is stubborn and doesn't lose weight quickly, then that's something I best neutralize if I want the opposite to be true. If we asked a child of divorced parents and another child with parents who are in a happy and healthy relationship to write down all their thoughts on marriage, we would likely get two very different stories, and these beliefs will undoubtedly affect how they proceed in their future relationships.

The deepest level of thought, the kind of story that takes a good bit of digging to uncover and some real deep work to heal, is a *core belief.* This is a belief that is so unconscious, you may not even realize you are operating from this place. Not only do you see the world through the lens of this skewed reality, but this belief also creates your identity and sets the foundation for all your other thoughts. Most likely this core belief was created in childhood or at a time of high positive emotion or negative trauma.

Brenda's parents divorced when she was twelve years old. The stress of the divorce, in conjunction with the onset of puberty, caused

Brenda to gain about thirty pounds. Her father noticed her weight gain and started telling her how gross she looked, how no guy would ever marry her unless she was skinny, and worst of all, that she would never be successful if she didn't lose the weight. This message at a young age, during the most traumatic time of Brenda's life, created a core belief that she would never be good enough. How did this bubble to the surface? Brenda became a high-functioning perfectionist, outwardly proving to everyone how "enough" she was. A switch had flipped in Brenda's brain, and from that point on striving to be perfect was her preferred method for trying to erase this feeling of lack. This perfectionist drive gave Brenda constant anxiety, which caused her to overeat. By the time she was thirty-five, she was married, she weighed 245 pounds, and she was the top performer in her real estate firm.

After working with Brenda for a few sessions, I helped her uncover her most limiting core belief. She was successful in all aspects of her life except for her weight. When it came to even the simplest of health improvements, Brenda would sabotage herself every time. She realized that by keeping the weight on she was proving her father wrong. Her size was saying, "Screw you, Dad. I'm fat, and I found love. I'm making a lot of money, and everyone likes me. You were wrong." Subconsciously she was equating weight loss and her father being right. Even though she wanted to take the weight off, her number one goal was to prove her father wrong. It was the only way she knew how to reject that nasty core belief of not being enough.

Unearthing destructive core beliefs and healing them at the root is how we free ourselves from the fiction of our lives and from negative beliefs about our weight. Now is a good time to pause and ask yourself the following questions:

1. What core beliefs do I have about my weight or my ability to follow through with my health goals?
2. Are there any theories I have mistaken for facts that, if rewritten, would help me feel healthier and happier?

To change our eating behaviors, we need to start by taking a good, hard look at our belief systems around food, our bodies, and what part of ourselves we are bringing to the weight-loss table. Your body is the product of your thoughts and beliefs. If you want permanent change, you have to train the mind with a new set of beliefs.

What Are Your Beliefs?

Many of your day-to-day thoughts stem from a deeper, more subconscious belief system. Your core beliefs shape who you imagine yourself to be and help you make sense of the world you live in. These deeply ingrained theories take form as you grow. They are shaped by your experiences, your environment, your life events, and the people who influence you.

Since our lives take very different paths, each of us will have different beliefs and identities (who we think we are). The one common thread is that each of us has a survival-trained mind. As mentioned earlier, this mind is meant to protect us by bringing to our attention everything that is wrong or could go wrong. Yet we grow up with basic beliefs that don't protect us or help us to survive. You could see how at one point they would have served us (think primal era: running from a bear, seeking shelter, finding food) but in current times are causing us much stress and harm. "I am not enough. I can't depend on anyone. The world is unsafe, and people are out to get me. Life is unfair. I have to make everything in my life happen. I have no help."

The most powerful influence on the human mind is our core beliefs about our identity, who we think we are. If you have a core belief that you are lazy or that the world is out to get you, no matter how much you try to be more productive or to feel safer in this world, you will sabotage your efforts to align with your core belief. How do you heal this? Start by asking yourself, *What do I want to believe?* Once you've discerned these new empowering beliefs, do the work to prove these beliefs to be true, using your own life experiences and the experiences of others. Remember, you see what you want to see.

Create a New Narrative

The more you control the voice in your head, the easier it will be to allow guidance to come forth from your higher self. If your house is dilapidated and built on a crooked foundation yet located on a beautiful piece of property, do you try to put up new walls, give the house a fresh coat of paint, and hope for the best? No. You tear that sucker to the ground. Strip it of everything, including the foundation, and then start from scratch. We need to break the mind down to its core beliefs, decide how we want to view the world, and then build up from there. This requires a new set of basic beliefs, a new system for you to honor and practice.

During my many years of working with clients and walking my own spiritual path, the following five core beliefs have helped me live in a more peaceful and meaningful way. Whether you love these five or wish to make up your own, I encourage you to print them out and put them in a place that allows you to see them throughout the day.

Five Core Beliefs

1. Everything happens *for* me, not *to* me. There is meaning and growth opportunity in this experience.
2. Everything is unfolding perfectly at the exact right time.
3. Out of this, *only good* will come.
4. The Universe is looking out for me and conspiring in my favor.
5. I am enough, and I am loved.

Let's examine these one at a time.

1. **Everything happens *for* me, not *to* me. There is meaning and growth opportunity in this experience.** You

can't control what happens in your life. Believe me, I've tried this from all angles (and endured a lot of suffering from doing so). You can, however, control what these events mean to you. You have the power to create any story you want. You can say, "This is the worst thing that has ever happened to me," or you can create a more positive and empowering narrative.

2. **Everything is unfolding perfectly at the exact right time.** We live in a time when the world is at our fingertips. Social media shows us the highlight reel of everyone's life, not the outtakes. One scroll through your Instagram feed, and you feel behind. "I should have a boyfriend / girlfriend / better job / child / more money / bigger home / bigger career / flatter stomach." Believing that everything is unfolding perfectly on your life path allows you to take a deep breath and be grateful for the way that your story is unfolding. You must trust that the person you look up to was at one time standing right where you are. There is nothing amiss here. This is *your* story, and it gets more beautiful once you surrender to it. Fries won't make you feel better about where you are in your life's path, but this belief will.
3. **Out of this, *only good* will come.** You are most likely in the habit of living your life in hindsight. You experience massive stress and emotional turmoil when something undesirable happens, and then years later you look back and say, "I understand why that happened." Think about your first heartbreak. Were you completely lovesick, devastated, and hopeless about ever finding love again? How do you feel about it now that some time has passed? Bad things are going to happen. It's simply the human experience. No one is exempt from the pitfalls of being alive. Imagine

being in the moment when the shit hits the fan and telling yourself that *only good will come of this*. This belief allows you to feel at peace, even while you are in the midst of chaos.

4. **The Universe is looking out for me and conspiring in my favor.** Whether you call it the Universe, God, Love, and so on, something more significant is guiding you and knows even better than you what you need to experience in your lifetime. Personally, I don't want to believe that it's all up to me. That's just too much pressure! I have peace knowing something greater is working its magic on my behalf.
5. **I am enough, and I am loved.** You don't have to be anything other than what you are right now. You don't have to be richer, thinner, smarter, or more successful. You will feel most fulfilled when you wake up every morning with the desire to be better than who you were the day before. The difference is the energy you bring to this appetite for more. Wanting to evolve as you come from a place of feeling enough has exponentially more power than wanting to be more to prove to yourself that you *are* enough.

When beginning to take control of the voice in your head, please be patient. Your first reaction will be to go to your default survival mind. Take a little space, and start to do the work. Call on your new belief system, and ask your higher self for guidance. Have compassion for yourself in the process; you are doing the hard work of rewiring yourself from a place of fear and control to one of love and surrender. This requires daily practice but will ultimately give you the clarity you need to take action and live your life's purpose. This purpose is nothing more than awakening to your gift and sharing it with the world, living in harmony with the flow of life, and enjoying your adventure as it unfolds.

Find Your Clarity

Once you begin to question the validity of what you think, you can start to separate from the monkey mind and allow your true self to shine through. From this place, you can create a clear vision for what you desire instead of being stuck in a story about what you can't achieve. With clarity on your side, you can say that you are not willing to give up what you want *most* (energy, confidence, strength) for what you want *right now* (food, comfort, instant gratification). By becoming vulnerable enough to explore your beliefs about your body and food, you start the journey of setting yourself free.

"I have to go see an energy healer" is not a sentence that used to fly out of my mouth. I was raised on Staten Island, after all, and my spiritual journey began much later in life. But I was desperate. I was going through the worst breakup of my life. I couldn't eat (which you know for me means that something very serious is happening), I couldn't sleep, and I was devastated. Therapy was helping, but it wasn't quick enough. It had been six months, and I was still reading old email exchanges and stalking my ex's Facebook page. I became addicted to the pain, and as much as I wanted to move on, I didn't want to let go of him, so I was stuck obsessing about what went wrong.

As I was replaying the drama to a friend of mine, who by that point was probably wishing I had lost her phone number, she interrupted me by offering the name of her mother's energy healer. I thought that as weird as it sounded, nothing could possibly make me feel worse, so I made an appointment with Steve the energy healer and hoped for the best. (The "best" being that somehow his magical powers would ship "you know who" to an island with all my other ex-boyfriends. In fact, shipping them all to Staten Island would be the perfect karmic torture.)

The appointment with Steve was mostly uneventful. I sat on a chair while he moved his hands over me in Reiki-type fashion. It wasn't until the end of the appointment that things started to get interesting. As I was getting ready to leave, he told me he had some homework for me. He said, "I want you to make a list of everything you want in a partner. I want you to be completely selfish and judgmental. Pretend the Universe is going to wave a magic wand and give you everything on that list. Please be thorough." Now, this was going to be a cinch for me. Be judgmental? Not a problem! No one had ever permitted me just to say what I wanted without putting a filter on it.

Although I no longer have that piece of paper, I do remember the funniest things I wrote down. Here are a few of them:

- He rubs my feet without asking me to rub his.
- He likes to play sports but doesn't watch them on TV.
- His mother is totally cool and not one of those annoying mothers-in-law you daydream about poisoning at Thanksgiving dinner.
- He lives a life without disease and dies in his sleep of natural causes only after I die minutes before him in a *The Notebook*–type scenario.

Of course, I had the typical "has to be kind, spiritually advanced, patient, successful, healthy, positive, nonreactive, loving, playful, hot body, great in bed" list of perfect-partner desires. It was so freeing to just put it all out there without censoring myself or allowing my mind to tell me a story of why I would never find this person.

Steve told me to bring the paper with me to our next session. I was so proud to show him my long list. I was a good student, judgmental and picky, just like he requested! I sat down and excitedly handed him the paper. I imagined he would burn it in some type of shamanic ceremony, and then I would roll it into a joint and smoke it, and all my wishes would come true.

Without looking at it, he turned it around so the words on the page faced me, and he said, "Are you all these things?" He then ripped up the paper and told me to take the next few months to work on getting myself to a place where that type of guy would be my vibrational match. If I wanted someone who was kind, patient, and playful, then I needed to practice being those things as well. If I wanted a guy with a hot body, then I needed to start taking care of myself again. Steve's Jedi mind trick worked. He gave me extreme clarity not only about the kind of person I wanted to be with but about the kind of person I wanted to be. Although we won't get to manifestation until chapter 9, I want to let you know right now that eight years later I married a man who rubs my feet almost every night without ever asking me to rub his in return. He's an avid cyclist but never watches sports on television, and I love his mother; she is the coolest mother-in-law you could ask for.

Before you attempt to achieve anything, *you must start by having extreme clarity about the outcome you want to create.* One of the best questions you can ask yourself before starting anything new, even a conversation, is, "What is my outcome? Why is this so important? What becomes available to me if I achieve this? What is withheld from me if I don't?"

Since you are reading this book, chances are that this is not the first time you have tried to lose weight. By now you have a theory that for you losing weight is too hard, maybe even impossible. After falling off the horse so many times with our failed diet attempts, we aren't super excited to jump back on, knowing that we might fall off and get hurt once again. We focus too much on the problem and not enough on the solution. Having clarity about what you want will keep your attention going in the right direction. Where you put your attention is where you manifest your reality. Do you think more about what you want than what you don't want? Do you look in the mirror and see the possibility or the failure?

Using clarity to stay focused on the outcome is integral to your long-term success. If you aren't anchored to the outcome at all times, you will ultimately drown in the process. The process of achieving anything worthwhile is going to be difficult. Think of three things that are massively important to you that you want to achieve. Now think about the process of getting there, the blood, sweat, and tears it will take to get you to the finish line. Are you motivated to act? No way, José. Take a deep breath and begin to visualize your outcome. Think about how it will feel to be at the end goal. Visualize what it will look like, the emotions you will experience, how your life will improve. Feeling more motivated? Having a clear outcome for your health journey is one of the most important aspects of your new path. You must remain focused on the outcome to be successful.

Before you sit down to write your clear vision for optimal health, make sure you are in the right state of mind. Jump around to some music, go for a jog around the block, jump on a trampoline, or move your body in a way that feels good. In other words, shake out your willies and any negative energy living in the body so that you are a clear vessel for writing. When you write, make sure to be as detailed as possible. If your vision is of you walking down the beach in a bikini, paint the picture on paper. What color is your bathing suit? Is your hair up or down? Is the sun shining, or is it sunset? How do you feel as you walk? What did you do for a workout that day, and what were your meals? If you were to read this vision to a stranger, he or she would be able to throw it onto a movie screen and have it play like the trailer of your future fabulous life.

Once you've written this vision, keep it somewhere close because you will be reading it every morning before you start your day. This image is what you want *most*. There's another aspect of desire, which is what you want right at the moment, and the two visions usually don't match up. What I want most may be to meditate every day to achieve a calm and peaceful inner self. What I want right now is to skip the meditations so I can knock some things off of my to-do list. What you want most is to wake up early and get to that exercise class. What you want right now may be to press snooze and try to get back to that dream where you are starring in *Fifty Shades of Grey*.

When I find myself in this predicament, I make this simple but powerful statement: *"I am not willing to give up what I want most for what I want right now."* When I say the words *what I want most*, I think about the vision I read that morning. It empowers me to get through the moment of instant gratification and reach deeper and more powerful goals. Say the outcome I want is to adopt healthier eating habits. I'm at a Mexican restaurant thinking this mantra over and over again as I sit in front of a basket of chips. Then I ask the waiter for guacamole with fresh-cut veggies and repeat my mantra. I wake up the next morning ecstatic that I made the best decision for the outcome that is most important to me. This doesn't always work, and when it doesn't, there is a deeper lesson for me to learn. Be gentle with yourself as you use this tool. There's always something to learn, and you are still moving forward on the path, whether or not it feels that way.

Skimmer's Delight

- ✓ We think up to sixty-five thousand thoughts a day — and most of them are negative and based on illusion, not truth.
- ✓ When you can start to separate story from fact, you empower yourself to choose higher-vibration thoughts (and then to crave higher-vibration foods). This practice allows you to eat well without needing a diet to keep you in line.
- ✓ You need clarity to say you are not willing to give up what you want most for what you want right now.
- ✓ You are worthy simply because you beat out all those other sperm-and-egg pairs. You don't need another reason.
- ✓ Take back control of your mind, and create new core beliefs that allow you to authentically desire health and wellness.
- ✓ If you focus on the process of what it takes to achieve your goal, you will fail. To be successful, you must remain focused on the outcome.

Make It Stick

1. Time to get crystal clear on paper. What do you want most? Write down your vision of optimal health, and use the following guidelines:

    - Use the present tense.
    - Write without fear.
    - Be as detailed as possible.
    - Explain why you want this (the "why" comes before the "how").

    Ask yourself, "What is my outcome? Why is this so important? What becomes available to me if I achieve this? What is withheld from me if I don't?"

2. Write your response to the following questions:

    - What core beliefs do I have about my weight or my ability to follow through with my health goals?
    - Are there any theories I have mistaken for facts that, if rewritten, would help me feel healthier and happier?
    - What do I *want* to believe about my body and my health?

3. Think about a major event in your life. How did this shape the way you now see the world? Did this event create a positive or negative belief? Without this belief, how would your life or actions be different today?
4. Journal about a time in your life when something happened and, in the moment, you completely resisted it (a breakup, a job change). Now that time has passed, explain why you think the Universe had your back. How did it show up for you in a way that you couldn't see at the time?

chapter 3

DIVINE PLEASURE AND EXQUISITE PAIN

When I buy cookies I eat just four and throw the rest away. But first I spray them with Raid so I won't dig them out of the garbage later. Be careful, though, because Raid really doesn't taste that bad.
— Janette Barber

If dieting were a sport, do you know who would be the most highly revered athlete of all time? A woman planning her dream wedding. A bride with a countdown to her final dress fitting? Watch out for that savage! She will do anything for the last spot in a spin class. If there's one premade salad left at Whole Foods, and both you and she are reaching for it, don't make direct eye contact, or better yet, bow to her and slowly back away. What is it about that dress and those wedding photos that completely converts the weak-willed into Hercules?

All our behaviors around food stem from our most basic emotional associations: pain and pleasure. We feel hundreds of emotions daily: happiness, boredom, fear, apathy, anger, surprise, sadness, nervousness, and the list goes on. As a survival technique, the primordial mind interprets these emotions to figure out whether we need to fight or flee. To simplify this crucial survival mechanism, the mind categorizes all our emotions as either feelings that cause pain or feelings that cause pleasure. Every thought, and simultaneous emotion that comes with it, triggers your survival mind to think, "Does this cause me pain (fight-or-flight) or does this cause me pleasure (create a habit)?"

Survival has set us up to be pleasure-seeking and pain-avoiding human beings. We run from the bear because being eaten would be painful and pretty inconvenient. We don't touch the fire because getting burned would cause us pain. Survival is in the here and now. The problem with this is that the mind is not taking into account non-life-threatening situations. In these cases, the long-term pleasure of not eating the cookie (weight loss, health, confidence) would serve us best, not the avoidance of the short-term pain of having to sit there craving it and not giving in.

Going to a restaurant and ordering a salad while everyone else at the table is chowing down on a shared appetizer of nachos and fries, let's face it, is (short-term) painful. Sitting there and waiting for your salad and not giving in to the (short-term) pleasure of how amazing that food will taste sucks. It causes (short-term) massive discomfort or, as the mind sees it, pain. Walking out of the restaurant feeling amazing, having enjoyed your salad and feeling extremely proud of yourself for staying true to your goals, creates long-term pleasure. A week later, going to the mall to try on clothes and feeling great because you are down five pounds provides even more long-term pleasure. Long-term pleasure keeps giving back. Short-term pleasure, also known as the four minutes of bliss we have when eating crappy food, comes with hefty long-term painful consequences.

The woman anticipating her wedding photos turns into Hercules for one very simple reason. If she doesn't love how she looks in her dress, every time she sees those wedding pictures, she will be in a massive amount of emotional pain. This is way more painful than saying no to sugar-laden foods in the moment. *We will avoid whatever causes more pain than pleasure.* The day after her wedding the possible pain of not looking good completely disappears. It's over, what's done is done. She will then go back to her default mode, and since she's been restricting herself for so long, the thought of giving in to instant gratification is simply too appealing.

Pleasure Comes with Pain

There's no way around it: most of our long-term pleasure will be attached to some amount of short-term pain. Feeling toned in your body is worth the time it takes to work out, the physical pain of feeling sore, and of course the most painful, ruining your beautiful blowout with all that sweat. Having money saved up in your bank account likely means that you endured some short-term pain of saying no to those fantastic shoes you saw in Nordstrom (but didn't need). Having a healthy and mutually respectful relationship means that you have experienced the short-term pain of feeling reactive (that's therapist talk for wanting to rip your partner's head off) but listening with an open heart and using loving words instead. Think about any aspect of your life in which you receive long-term pleasure. You should immediately be able to recognize the sacrifice, or short-term pain, you are willing to endure to receive what you have your heart set on.

Short-term pleasure comes with its own set of consequences. Giving in to the craving of the moment means you are going to feel it later. Drunk-texting your ex and waking up to the embarrassment the next day...and the days and weeks after that. Staying up too late to watch television and skipping your workouts the rest of the week because you kept pressing the dreaded snooze button. Putting those cute sneakers on your charge card and then having constant anxiety about money. Drinking too much because, in the moment, you are having the best time, only to feel terrible the whole next day and not ever being able to reach your weight-loss goals. Not flossing because it's annoying and then having extensive dental work years later. What you will notice about short-term pleasure is just that...it's short. It's deceptively attractive in the moment, but take a step back and see it for what it is. Ask yourself if it is ever truly worth it in the long run. So why do we choose it time after time? When are we going to learn our lesson?

Now, don't make that face of defeat! This isn't your fault. We are hardwired to seek pleasure and avoid pain. When survival was our utmost directive, this served us well, but our choices are no longer find shelter or die; they're eating chips and guacamole or abstaining. If you want to master the game of permanent weight loss, you will need to learn how to reprogram your pain and pleasure associations.

The Most Common Types of Pain

Since we all experience monkey mind, we all share the same pain stories. They are mainly concerned with our lack of resources (time, money, and other people) or merely with the fact that we want what we want when we want it. We are in the habit of giving into the pleasure of the moment, and we don't yet have the tools to override that deeply ingrained pattern.

The most common gripe I hear about weight loss and health is the lack of time. We don't have time to cook, we don't have time to work out, we don't have time to go food shopping, and we certainly don't have time to meditate. There are simply not enough hours in the day.

A few years back when I was studying the work of Deepak Chopra, I came across a documentary that portrayed his daily life. In that film, Deepak mentioned that he wakes up in the middle of the night, meditates for four or so hours, and then begins his day, running multiple businesses. At that moment I realized that what we accomplish has nothing to do with time. The reason is never that we don't have time. *Bottom line: we make time for the things that are important to us.* I'm not saying that meditation should be more important than sleep; I'm just asking you to take a hard look at what you spend your time on. Whatever you spend your time on is what's most important to you. Are you consciously making this decision?

There have been plenty of days when my story was that I didn't have time to do a twenty-minute meditation or a twenty-minute workout. In that same day, I watched two of my favorite television shows and spent at least twenty minutes throughout the day on social media. Perhaps I've even spent the time doing something "productive" like cleaning the house, so I'm under the impression that I wasn't goofing off. What will I remember fifty years from now — the fact that my floor was always clean or that I worked toward a level of health that ensured I lived to see my grandchildren graduate from high school? It always humbles me when I go on vacation and don't watch television the entire week. The best part is that I don't care! Those people and story lines are suddenly so unimportant to me. I'm immersed in the world, in the present moment, in discovering the new. Then as soon as I get home and back into the work grind, those shows once again become my nightly saving grace. We have to sit down with clarity and decide how we are going to spend our days, or else the days will happen *to* us, and the result is not one that will ultimately fulfill us.

Can you see a correlation to food? Have you had the experience of going on vacation to a new place and being fulfilled by new people and experiences; and while you may enjoy your meals, the rest of the day you aren't thinking about food? You are so fulfilled by the pleasure of life's adventures that you don't need to fill that void with mashed potatoes. Once you come home and jump back onto the Monday-through-Friday hamster wheel, all of a sudden the only thing that will make you happy is a milkshake and a Julia Roberts movie (am I projecting?).

This point is so important that it warrants repeating. There is no such thing as *not* having enough time. You make time for the things that are important to you. It's time for you to ask yourself, "What is truly important to me?" Get out of the unconscious cycle and think about the long-term pleasure and what is truly at stake.

The second and third runners-up are pain stories about money and the lack of support from other people. "Organic food is too expensive. I really need a trainer to stay motivated, but I can't afford one. I need to hire a babysitter if I'm going to exercise or cook, and I can't afford it. I don't have anyone around to help me watch my children or to help me cook and clean." I know how true all this can feel in the moment. I get stuck all the time in stories I don't even realize aren't my actual reality. Just know they are all stories made up by the uncreative mind.

The second you say something with absolute conviction, question the validity of it. The mind loves to live in absolutes. Remember, a fact can't be changed, but a story has room for creativity. Just this morning when I woke up, my mind said to me, "You don't have time for meditation today." I happened to get to the office five minutes earlier than planned, so I sat in my car and closed my eyes. It may not have been the twenty minutes on the couch that I'm used to, but I made it happen only because I changed my story from "I don't have time to do it the way I'm supposed to" to "a five-minute meditation is better than a twenty-minute meditation that doesn't happen." As soon as you change your language around these limiting beliefs, you can turn these painful associations into pleasurable opportunities. In other words, you can scramble your pain and pleasure pathways.

By now you understand why you avoid certain things that are good for you and repeatedly do other things that are not so good for you. It's not because you are lazy or have no willpower. You're just telling yourself inaccurate stories about what is painful and pleasurable in your life, and these stories are playing out to contradict your new positive core beliefs. I don't just want you to power through and do the right thing. As long as you associate pain with healthy behaviors, no amount of willpower will create permanent change. You have to do some mental digging and create new pleasurable stories around your most important healthful behaviors.

The Resistance

I am happiest when I am writing. It is my most creative outlet. Do you know what I do right before I sit down and write? Anything and everything possible, just so I don't have to start. I'll do some pretty painful things, like cleaning the kitty litter box or emptying the dishwasher; I'll even call my grandparents and let them complain to me about why I moved so far away from them and ruined their lives. I'll pluck my chin hair (I promised you full disclosure) or change my sheets, and if I could, I'd cut the grass in my backyard blade by blade with scissors. If you find yourself doing the same kinds of thing, you are in good company. Finally, when there is nothing left for me to do, I'll sit down and start writing. About ten seconds in, I start feeling fantastic. The whole morning I carry around the weight of procrastination, and the second I start writing I feel like a million bucks.

What is this constant resistance we face when trying to do the right thing? It's simply a scrambled pain and pleasure pathway. Regard resistance as an invisible evil, showing up in the exact place where your deepest work is to be done. I'm sure you meet resistance when it is time to do all the things you need to do to live your best possible life. Why is this the case? Because *we have false stories about how things make us feel.* I am subconsciously telling myself that writing is painful, and you are telling yourself that losing weight and feeling free in your body is more painful than staying in the hell you are in right now (if ever there was a hell, hating the body you have and obsessing about food is it). Time to straighten these emotions out once and for all!

So, how did I get myself to sit down and write this book? As soon as I woke up, I told myself the stories I needed to hear. I told myself how much I love writing and how accomplished I feel, and I imagined how many people this book will help. I attached even more pleasure by making myself a fun little writing setup, playing music, lighting a candle, placing energy-increasing crystals all around myself like an altar, sitting outside and writing while my cats play and I watch the leaves falling from the tree. I set myself goals that feel really pleasurable to achieve, and I cheerleaded myself the whole way through.

I attach the same formula to everything regarding my health. When it comes to working out, I think about what is most pleasurable to me. I need cute workout clothes, good music, and a preplanned workout routine that doesn't take more than thirty minutes, and I need to get it done first thing in the morning. When I cook, I watch Netflix, and I time myself because it's fun for me to say that I spent an hour and a half in the kitchen and made myself clean food for the next three days. When I wash the dishes, I listen to a fluff podcast about the latest celebrity gossip, or I call a girlfriend; okay, that's a lie. I never wash dishes, not with this perfect mani (that's what my husband is for). Throughout the process, I use a mantra that reminds me of the long-term pleasure of it all.

Before you jump into the next chapter, I want you to put this book down and make a list of the top three actions you know would yield the most benefit for your health. I want you to make a list of all the pain (which will be all short-term), and then make a twice-as-long list of the long-term pleasures. One by one, I want you to cross out each item on your pain list by creating another story around it. You won't be able to cross out everything (cleaning the litter box is nasty, and there's no way around that), but I want you to get your pain list down to two to three items, max. Look at the two lists and decide to step into action. Decide to tell yourself a new story about pain and pleasure. What will you do tomorrow to follow through with this new way of thinking?

Skimmer's Delight

- ✓ We are wired to avoid pain and seek pleasure in the here and now; the brain doesn't think long-term.
- ✓ You need to consider the long-term pleasure of behaviors, not just the short-term pain.
- ✓ If you want to stop doing something (overeating, for example) to reach the next level of health, you need to attach more pain to it than pleasure.
- ✓ If you want to start doing something to reach the next level of health (exercising, meditating, cooking), you need to attach more pleasure to doing it and more pain to not doing it.
- ✓ Resistance is an invisible evil, showing up in the exact place where your deepest work is to be done.
- ✓ Kick resistance's ass by showing up like you are getting paid.

Make It Stick

1. Journal about three things you need to be doing right now to achieve your vision of optimal health (but have been inconsistent with). Separate a page by making four quadrants (see example on next page). Label the boxes: short-term pain of doing it, long-term pleasure of doing it, long-term pain of not doing it, short-term pleasure of not doing it. See which column creates most long-lasting happiness.
2. What are three things you can do to ensure this behavior gets completed?

COOKING

SHORT-TERM PAIN OF COOKING	LONG-TERM PLEASURE OF COOKING
takes time	feeling healthy
have to clean up	losing weight
	living longer
	having glowing skin
	having tons of energy
	feeling proud of myself
	saving money

LONG-TERM PAIN OF NOT COOKING	SHORT-TERM PLEASURE OF NOT COOKING
less money in the bank	more free time
never lose the weight	don't have to clean up
less confidence	more social to eat out
low-quality foods	
cancer risk	
overeating	
less energy	

chapter 4

IS STRESS STRESSING YOU OUT?

I am an old man and have known a great many troubles,
but most of them never happened. — **Mark Twain**

The greatest weapon against stress is our ability
to choose one thought over another. — **William James**

When I asked my client Ruby what she thought her trigger was for her on-and-off dieting, she said, "Honestly, when everything in my life is going well, it's really easy for me to eat healthily. I don't know why, but everything seems to fall into place. The second something happens that I'm not expecting, my exercise and healthy eating fly out the window. It's like I can't manage the stress and my health at the same time." Ruby, I feel you, girlfriend. This is exactly why stress elimination is an integral part of permanent weight loss and overall health and happiness.

Before I teach you how to see stress for what it is (the antithesis of present-moment awareness and a real happiness buzzkill), let's differentiate between the two types of stress in your life. *Eustress* is defined as "a positive form of stress having a beneficial effect on health, motivation, performance, and emotional well-being." It's the stress you feel preparing for a project you are truly excited about or the last-minute rush of getting yourself ready for an upcoming vacation or adventure. This mental push increases your output, feels exciting, and brings you to the next level of growth and performance capability. *Distress*, or most commonly what we refer to simply as "stress," causes anxiety, feels incredibly unpleasant, decreases your performance, and leaves you feeling frozen in fear.

For the remainder of this book, when I talk about stress I'm referring to distress, the negative thinking that we can all eliminate. It's for this reason that I never liked the term *stress management*. I don't want to manage it; I want tools to help me eliminate it from my life! Sounds impossible, but I promise you that if a man can land on the moon and the Kardashians can solve world hunger one lip kit at a time, then I can show you how to kick stress's ass once and for all.

Stress Redefined

The first step to eliminating stress from your life (and the inches from your waistline caused by stress eating) is to see it for what it truly is: fear. *Stress* is a code word for *fear*. When you feel fear, you have officially left the present moment and are off in some future horrible alternative universe where bad things happen. Take school, for example (or work, money, relationships: they all apply). Remember being stressed-out about finals week or that colossal paper due at the end of the semester? It wasn't the tests or papers themselves that were causing you stress. It was the fear of not being prepared to do well enough that caused it. In that moment of self-doubt and worry, your stress was projecting the negative outcome of an event (failing) that did not yet happen. You could have been putting all that negative energy into studying and preparing, but instead you were wasting your time focusing on what you didn't want to have happen.

Most of the things you stress about are not happening in real time. In fact, if any of these things actually did happen, you would find yourself better equipped to deal with them than you think. It is your mind's sadistic imagination that plagues you day to day. In her incredible book *The Fear Cure*, Lissa Rankin explains, "Most of the fears that plague us today exist only in our imagination. They are not real threats, but the amygdala in the primordial brain can't tell the difference, so the nervous system gets stuck in unnecessary stress responses." In other words, your body perceives the stress as happening, so you physically react even though you are not experiencing anything close to the story you have created in your mind.

What if your negative story manifested and you did, in fact, wind up failing your final exams? It was disappointing to see those grades, but what's done is done. You can choose between learning from it and moving forward on the search for better studying tools and allowing this experience to create an identity for you about not being smart enough. If you chose the latter, you would enter the stress cycle once more, worrying about what those grades would mean for getting into graduate school or whether or not they would affect your ability to get a good job. Notice the pattern of stress. It clouds your opportunity in the present moment to empower the true peace of mind and the mentality of acceptance that we all desire.

Why does the mind torture us this way? *Our survival mind believes that the only way to be safe is to be afraid.* Since we don't want to admit we are walking around in fear all day long, we use the word *stress* because our society accepts this state of being as a cultural norm. Oh, you're stressed? Join the club, or better yet, eat a club sandwich with chips; that will make your stress melt away. I want to challenge you to completely remove the word *stress* from your vocabulary and replace it with the word *fear*. Doing this will trigger you to do the internal work to turn your story around. Then fear will carry a beautiful message that it's time to get out of your head and back into your heart.

Your new challenge will look something like this. You don't need the help of a coach to get out of stress; just picture having this conversation with yourself. Here I'm taking the role of your "higher self."

Me: Hey, you, what's up? You seem a little frazzled.

You: Ugh, I'm totally stressed-out about wearing a bathing suit at my friend's pool party this weekend.

Me: Try replacing the term *stressed-out* with *fearful*. What is it you fear?

You: I guess I'm scared people are going to judge me. I feel bad enough when I look in the mirror; I don't need anyone to notice every dimple on my thighs.

Me: Well, sounds like you are the only one judging you right at this moment. These people are your friends, no? They will love and accept you for who you are. And if someone is judging you, she is simply distracting herself from self-judgment. Notice that the more you judge yourself, the more you tend to judge other people.

You: That's true. I guess I am pretty judgmental of others, now that I think about it.

Me: That's because you spend a lot of the time judging yourself. Let me ask you: Will you be checking out the other women at the pool party and judging their bodies?

You: To be honest, yes. I'll be looking at them and trying to find someone who looks worse than me so I can feel better about myself. I'll also be jealous of the woman with the best-looking body.

Me: Does that say more about that woman's body or your insecurities? Since we know the answer to this, if someone else is judging you at the party, is that about you or them?

You: It's about them.

Me: Let's remove this fear (stress) by reframing your story. Give it a try. Replace "I'm so stressed about the pool party this weekend" with the opposite, more empowering thought.

You: "I'm looking forward to this party as an opportunity for me to accept where I am in my weight-loss journey and to practice not judging the other women there. I don't have to be self-conscious because I know that my body does not define who I am in my heart, and also I've been working on my weight loss and having success! I'm going to feel pumped about that."

Me: That's awesome! Let's add a mantra for you to repeat at the party to help center you when you get caught in your head. How does it feel to say, "I love and accept exactly the way I look right now, and I look forward to putting in the work to get my body in peak shape and health, where I deserve to be"?

You: That feels really good.

There is an old saying, "If you are depressed you are living in the past. If you are anxious, you are living in the future. If you are at peace, you are living in the present." Did you notice in this recent example that being judged in a bathing suit didn't even happen yet? Neither has that deadline you missed at work, that mistake you made, that plane that crashed, that fight you got into with your friend, that deal you missed out on closing and that guy/woman you never met.

Let's be honest; sometimes this shit *does* happen. You did make that mistake, or get fired, or worse. Your fear has manifested, and it's occurring in the present moment. Does that then make stress useful? No. One or all of the core beliefs I taught you in chapter 2 will come in very handy to help you surrender to whatever *is* and move forward as a wiser, more experienced version of yourself. As a reminder, here are those core beliefs again:

1. Everything happens *for* me, not *to* me. There is meaning and growth opportunity in this experience.
2. Everything is unfolding perfectly at the exact right time.
3. Out of this, *only good* will come.
4. The Universe is looking out for me and is conspiring in my favor.
5. I am enough, and I am loved.

The Three Ways We Get into Stress

My husband and I dated on and off for five years until we decided to get hitched. At the time we got engaged, we had already been living together for two years. Other than the pretty ring on my finger and a wedding to plan, we pretty much went about our lives as usual. Not much changed except one very disturbing thought pattern. I started obsessively worrying about my husband-to-be dying and leaving me a widow. I would stare at this man sleeping beside me and conjure up all the horrible things that could happen to him, leaving me heartbroken and ruining my life forever. I pictured myself not being able to work or eat; my sister would have to come over and feed me or else I would waste away from a broken heart. You would think I had a lot of free time on my hands, but no, the mind decided this would be a great use of what little downtime I had with my fiancé.

There must have been something about that next level of commitment that triggered this stress/fear response. The added vulnerability of choosing this wonderful man as my life partner made it crystal clear that someone besides me could change the course of my life forever. I no longer felt in control of my emotions. While I was busy ruminating, I didn't realize that I fell for the trap of one of the three ways we get into stress: *we focus on the things we can't control.*

As someone who has struggled most of her life with stress and anxiety, I realize that anxiety (stress, worry, fear) comes from the battle between our minds and our higher selves. Your higher self knows that most of what occurs in your life is out of your control. It tells you that the only thing in your power is how you react to these events. On a deeper level, you know that your happiness and peace of mind are directly related to how successful you are at reframing a negative event into an opportunity for growth. On the other hand, your mind tells you that the more you try to control life, the safer you will be. This battle between control and surrender creates chronic anxiety, heightened whenever something unexpected pops up in your life. Whenever I feel anxious I know I'm fighting against the ultimate truth: *the quality of my life is directly related to the amount of unknown I can comfortably make peace with.*

Focusing on what is out of your control will create suffering. Worrying about my husband dying before me doesn't do anything to keep him safe. In fact, it ruins my present moment. Instead of enjoying lying next to the man I love, I'm trying to protect myself from planning a funeral. I know this is a morbid topic, and I could easily have picked something else to drive this point home, but I want you to be brave enough to face your deepest fears to uncover your deepest truth. Surrendering to the present moment is the most powerful tool you have. Not wasting your time stressing about what you can't control frees up a lot of time to laugh, play, and enjoy the life you have worked so hard to create for yourself.

The second way we get into stress is that *we make things more important than they are.* Work deadlines, family drama, relationship issues, scheduling mishaps, traffic, delayed flights — think about the last five events that left you feeling completely frazzled. Did you, by any chance, make these events a teensy-weensy bit more important than they were in reality? What reality, you ask? The reality in which you go with the flow and live a stress-free life!

Last, we hypothesize the future worst-case scenario, or as Brené Brown beautifully states, "we dress-rehearse tragedy." As I've said before, fear is the projection into the future of a negative outcome, an outcome that has not yet happened and very probably will not happen (or if it did happen, you would find yourself handling it much better than you imagined). I find it sad that my mind can take something purely positive and ruin it by keeping me rooted in fear. I solidify the deal on that amazing hard-to-get speaking opportunity, and my mind says, "Great! Now, what if you mess it up?" I finish planning a beach vacation, and it's time to get excited, and the mind says, "Oh no, what if it rains the whole time?" What about you? You get that new job and then worry about performance. You finally get pregnant and then worry about the health of the baby. You meet the love of your life and then worry about whether he/she will stay faithful to you. You lose five pounds and then worry about the weight coming back on.

The great news is that as easy as it is to get into stress, it's just as easy to get out of it — not by eating our weight in chocolate peanut butter cups but by using our tools and having the mind work for us instead of against us. If we get into stress by focusing on what we can't control, making things more important than they are, and daynightmaring (I made up this word; it's a daydream you never intended to make real) worst-case scenarios, then we get out of stress by doing the opposite.

Next time you catch yourself focusing on something you can't control, ask yourself, "What about this situation *can* I control?" If my end-of-life plan (that my husband and I die in our sleep at the same moment while holding hands dreaming of soft-serve ice cream) doesn't pan out exactly how I'd hoped, the only piece of this that's in my control is how present and grateful I am for our time together right now. I will reframe this worry into gratitude and ask myself how I can enjoy even more the moments we share together now. I have to trust that whatever happens, it will happen *for* me, not *to* me.

Next time (and I guarantee that this will happen in the next thirty minutes) your mind tries to make something out to be more frightening, annoying, frustrating, and stressful than it is, see if you can make it even less important than it really is. Remind yourself that you will likely not care about this issue when you are eighty years old and in a rocking chair, surrounded by your beautiful grandchildren. You probably won't care about it in ten years, five years, one year, six months, or in some cases even one week.

Last, as you catch yourself conjuring up the worst-case scenario, do a quick and powerful turnaround. "What is the best-case scenario that could come from this? How can I keep my focus on this and make it happen?" Notice how you feel when you think about the best-case scenario. Now take one minute and go back to thinking about the worst possible outcome. How do you feel now? It's ultimately up to you.

Although I'm all for positive thinking, I do think it's wise to manage the downside. Your mind is going to go there anyway, so I figure if you think about it logically one time, then when your mind slips into worry you can calm it by reminding it that you've already managed the worst-case scenario. Take a moment and think about the downside of whatever you are focusing on. What will you do if the worst-case scenario does in fact come true? Make a plan, grab onto one of your new core beliefs for support, and know that going with the flow of life winds up rewarding you in ways you never imagined. And maybe you'll discover that the worst-case scenario isn't the end of the world after all.

Living a life filled with stress and worry not only makes you sick, but it also gives food an unnecessary and inappropriate amount of power, leading you to binge or restrict food to grasp some illusory sense of control. Deconstructing the illusion of stress guarantees us a better chance of staying in the now. Since the fundamental basis of health is present-moment awareness, eliminating stress is the best diet we could ever go on (and never go off).

Skimmer's Delight

✓ The end goal of all end goals is to be happy and at peace. If you don't feel happy, you are going to try to eat (and therefore diet) your way there. It won't work.

✓ Your plate is a reflection of your inner state.

✓ *Stress* is a code word for *fear* — and fear can't exist in the present moment when you practice surrendering.

✓ If you want to get out of stress, you must practice focusing only on the things you can control. You must make things less important than they appear, and daydream best-case scenarios into existence.

✓ Trust that the Universe is looking out for you and that everything is unfolding perfectly. It's all happening for your highest good.

Make It Stick

Write about something in your life right now that is causing you stress. Rework the statement to explain your fear, and use the tools in this chapter to arrive at an outcome that leaves you most at peace.

PART TWO

lose the weight

chapter 5

ONE SIZE FITS NO ONE (AND IT'S A LITTLE TIGHT IN THE CROTCH)

I tried every diet in the book. I tried some that weren't in the book. I tried eating the book. It tasted better than most of the diets.
— **Dolly Parton**

The word *diet* has become emotionally charged in our culture, especially if you have been on one, or a hundred of them, in your lifetime. The truth is that technically everyone's on a diet. Whether it's healthy food you're eating or processed junk, a diet is simply the food we are choosing to eat at the moment. Yet the word *diet* has always equaled *food prison* for me, since for years that's the only way I knew how to lose weight.

My mother always fed our family relatively healthy foods. I stayed very active as a young child and didn't focus on how I looked. It wasn't until puberty that I started gaining weight and becoming overly aware of just how imperfect my body seemed to be. Thus began my quest to try every single diet imaginable, only to fail time and time again.

In retrospect, it's pretty easy to see the central theme of each of my sad little failed attempts. I went *on* a diet, so the only next logical step was to go *off* of said diet and dive directly, face-first, into a bag of chips. I called this my "weekday-warrior" phase. As you know, during the week I cooked my meals, drank "dessert" tea at night, and counted down the moments until Friday. Food prison felt like the only acceptable option during the week, and on Friday I would break free and indulge in reckless abandonment.

By Sunday I would have eaten everything and anything I could get my hands on. As Sunday night came to a close, I grew more and more anxious, knowing that tomorrow I would wake up and have to repent for my late-night cookie crimes. Monday brought the mental shackles back again. Each week I could feel a little more self-loathing creeping in, and a little less trust that I could ever be happy in my body.

And as you also know, one day it hit me: what I was doing was not working. I know this epiphany seems obvious, but the mind has a very complicated way of thriving on negativity and keeping us stuck. The truth was simple; I didn't know what to eat for my body. I entertained constant cravings for crappy (but tasty) things, and I felt mentally and physically tired all the time. My digestive system was a wreck, and I was frustrated by the pointlessness of it all.

Here I'd like to pause and say that I'm not anti-diet. I'm also not pro-diet. Wait a second, are we dieting or are we not dieting?! Our culture is fighting decades of body shaming with an anti-diet body acceptance message. This message empowers women to simply love themselves at whatever size they are. This message quite often comes with the anti-diet mantra: "Fuck dieting; just love yourself!"

Self-love and acceptance is a fantastic message to spread. In fact, loving and accepting where you are is the only way to create change. Long-term change is never created by force; it can only grow from true self-love. As amazing as this sounds, it is not the end of the story. Yes, I want you to love yourself. I want you to love yourself so fiercely that you decide to demand more of yourself. Your mantra becomes: "I'm worth it. I'm going to show up for myself and start treating myself not just with loving words but with loving thoughts, actions, and movements.

My body is going to be a physical reflection of how much I love and support myself." This mantra is the foundation of your change. See the difference? If a special diet or workout regimen is what you need to truly love and respect what your body is asking for, then you have to shift your mind to get in alignment with this new plan.

So as not to beat around the bush, I believe we all need to be on individualized diets. There are just too many delicious, horrible-for-you foods out there that if we ate them every day would make us sick. We need to erect a set of loving boundaries around food. Since you know that our thoughts are the ultimate drivers of our dieting behaviors, you will agree with me that *dieting without spiritual tools is utter chaos.*

It took me years to realize that just because we *know* better doesn't mean we *do* better. Applied knowledge can be the most powerful tool you have, but knowledge alone will get you nowhere. I could have a PhD in nutrition and eat McDonald's for breakfast every day. It's what we *do* with the knowledge that changes our lives. Passion, applied knowledge, a deep desire for change, and a ton of self-compassion are the keys to transforming your life.

Diets Are Not the Devil

As I said above, I want to neutralize the word *diet.* If you eat, you are on a diet. We could be on a French fry diet (yum) or a grapefruit diet (yuck), but whether or not we know it, we all have a set of rules that governs what we put into our mouths. Ideally, you would be on the no-diet diet, and that's like the quiet guy at school whose lack of game is the best game in town. I want you to be the shy guy who gets all the dates. I call this the "I Can Eat Anything I Want, but I Mostly Choose to Eat Foods That Make Me Feel and Look Amazing" Diet.

Although we each have a unique set of nutritional needs, we all have one thing in common. We are all human, and therefore we all require the same nutritional foundation. This foundational nutrition protocol is to maintain a diet that minimizes sugar, alcohol, and foods that are chemically and artificially processed. Simply put, we should eat a majority of foods that rot and spoil quickly because that means they are living, and living foods make us feel alive! This is probably the only generalized statement I can make that applies to everyone, regardless of age, gender, and genetic history (no, wait, we should also meditate daily, practice patience and compassion, and be kind to ourselves and others). Now, perhaps you need to cut out dairy and grains, or beans, or eggs, or red meat. Or maybe you need to adjust your ratios of protein, carbs, and fat. Your unique medicine will require a period of trial and error, and I'll show you how to tweak this. In the back of this book I include a general baseline chart so you can see in detail the foods you want to maximize and the foods you want to stay the hell away from, except for when you are at a state fair. Then you should absolutely order the fried pizza.

Your healthy diet is not without a set of rules. Remember, everyone has rules about food, whether or not they know it. One person might have only one rule, which is that she eats whatever she wants. This may sound like wonderful food freedom, but when you eat whatever the mind tells you to, you will be feasting on food laden with the most addictive substances. This kind of freedom to eat whatever you want will make you feel trapped in a body that doesn't work right or look good. This type of food freedom creates body prison. A more enlightened way to look at food freedom is to use loving boundaries to feel free in your body, mind, and soul. With this mentality, it's not that I *can't* eat certain foods, it's that I *choose* to eat in a way that ultimately makes me feel free: free in my body, free to wear what I want, free with boundless energy, free to choose how I show up for myself every day.

Personally, I have an extremely sensitive digestive system. Because of this, I need a lot of rules around food to feel good (and to poop daily, which is a big communication from your body that you are putting the right foods into it). Whatever the case may be for you, the rule-following part of a diet will be much easier if you *stop associating rules with restriction* and you start thinking of rules as *loving boundaries* that help guide you at times when you feel out of sync with your higher self.

These loving boundaries are your friend. You will create them with my help; they will not be forced on you. You will create these boundaries to match your vision for optimal health. If you simply want to lose weight, you might have a rule to eat only what fits in a cereal bowl. If you want to poop every day, you may have to create a loving boundary around avoiding dairy and gluten.

You are not wrong to want that beach body or peak physical strength; you simply need to come to terms with the fact that these outcomes require more discipline and a stricter set of loving boundaries. If this is your goal, then your mind needs to shift your current definition of the word *moderation*. Regardless of your specific health goals, one of the most important shifts you can make is to stop attaching emotional pain to these guidelines and start thinking of them as your vehicle to ultimate health and happiness.

How We Became So Confused

Maybe I'm biased, but I don't know of any subject more contradictory than nutrition: "Beans can't be digested and therefore are inflammatory; don't touch them." "No, no, no. It's meat that causes cancer, and it rots in your stomach, go vegan!" "Beans and meat are fine; it's fat that you have to watch out for. I have studies to prove it!"

A few years back, I worked with a special client. She walked into my office and plopped down in front of me, visibly exhausted. Her skin had a grayish hue and was covered in acne. Her hair was falling out. She was about twenty-five pounds overweight, and she looked very sick. As I was listening to her and noticing her body's sign language (dull eyes, weak nails, coated tongue, inflamed skin), one of her tattoos caught my eye. On the side of her left arm, she had a tattoo that said "vegan."

"Oh, no," I thought to myself. "If I decide that this woman needs animal protein to heal her body, I'm going to have a hell of a time convincing someone who is so committed to her way of eating that she got it tattooed on her body!" *You have to be careful when the way you eat becomes part of your identity.* It may start as a noble and moral act, but before you know it, your mind gives it the power to define you as a person. As strong as this identity may be, with enough pain in your life, you will be willing to change anything to feel better. This woman was so depleted and miserable, she was willing to open her mind in order to let me help her heal.

When it comes to body imbalance, barring the extreme exception, healing occurs when you do the opposite of whatever you were doing to get you to the imbalance in the first place. I started her healing protocol by slowly introducing bone broth, with small servings of eggs and fish. Eventually, she started eating all kinds of animal protein, and within six weeks her hair started growing back, her energy restored itself, and she started losing weight. Years later, I ran into her at the grocery store, and she looked amazing. She joked with me that I should help her pay for her tattoo removal. Being the budget-savvy woman that I am, I told her we could save money simply by adding to it, making it "veganish."

I don't share this story to make vegan diets look bad. In fact, I'm positive that vegan diets have saved thousands of lives. I share it with the intention of conveying the ultimate truth about diets: different diet protocols work for different people. *One diet doesn't work for anyone all the time.* Your life changes, your body changes, and your food requirements change as well. The key is to learn how to listen to your body's communication so you can give it what it needs.

Whenever you encounter a topic around which there are two strong and opposing viewpoints, it is safe to automatically assume that both theories are simultaneously right and wrong. In the case of nutrition and nourishing your unique body, one size cannot possibly fit all. Someone becomes vegan, and it works wonders for her health. Then she thinks, "If it worked for me, it must work for everyone!" and she writes a book. It works for quite a few people, and then they create momentum, a following.

Simultaneously, another person tries cutting out grains and beans, calls it the paleo diet, and proclaims it to be the be-all and end-all of healthy eating. Because both these people are stuck in needing to be right, they search for all the studies that support their viewpoints. Repeat this cycle with absolutely every fad diet out there, and this is how we wind up in the health section of our local bookstore, completely overwhelmed and confused as to which dogma we should follow and why the heck there are so many out there in the first place.

I'm not going to pretend that I know exactly what you should eat at every meal, and neither should any other expert who doesn't know you personally. What I will share with you will allow you to pinpoint what you should be eating 95 percent of the time. The other 5 percent only your body can tell you. Tweaking your nutrition will come down to learning the signals of your body. I am truly teaching you how to become your own nutritionist and to transcend the diet dogma once and for all.

The Simplicity of Your Eating Foundation

I'm not going to do that bitchy thing where I write a book about losing weight but don't tell you what to eat in fear that doing so will activate food restriction, therefore defeating the purpose of the whole message. I get it; we need to understand *what* to eat as well as understanding *why* we eat, or don't eat, it. In the rest of this chapter, I'll put on my practitioner's hat and tell you how to eat to lose weight. This information won't, however, give you the slightest clue about how to keep it off. It will, however, lay the foundation so that you never again do the master cleanse to drop five pounds before a big Mexican vacation. I assure you that the rest of this book will teach you how to eat healthfully on a consistent basis and without those dreaded food shackles dragging you down.

Real Food vs. Fake Food

Do you find it weird that some foods in your pantry are years old? Not only have they been around for some time, but you could eat them right now, and they would taste the same way they did a year earlier. Food technology emerged as a way to solve public health problems, prevent deficiencies, and increase microbiological safety. We needed to make foods safer to eat, we needed to make them last longer, and we needed to make more food available for the masses. At the time these advancements came along, they were desperately needed. However, along the way, greed turned this science into a massive money-making machine of disease-causing Frankenfoods. Large corporations in charge of mass food production created chemical additives, fake fats, sugar substitutes, and artificial colors for foods that are not fit for human consumption.

Once we take the technology out of our food, we start following the energy principle of eating. The simple principle of energy exchange is this: humans are energy sources. We are a bunch of atoms bouncing off one another. To keep ourselves alive and energetic, we need to eat energy, much like a car needs fuel to run. Foods that are filled with energy in the form of vitamins, minerals, cofactors, and enzymes, are "alive" foods. The more alive and vital a particular food is, the quicker it is going to rot and spoil.

A vegetable will begin to wilt and lose its nutrition fairly quickly after being separated from its source (soil, light, and water). In contrast, boxed cereal can stay on the shelf for at least six months. The veggie is alive; the cereal is not. We feel dull when we eat processed, dead, shelf-stable foods. We feel alive and vital when we eat unprocessed foods that come from the earth. The farther away a food gets from its true source, the more processed and dead it becomes. An apple is a living food. Apple juice and apple fruit leather are not.

Our relationship with food is very layered. Yet this aspect of eating, or knowing *what to eat*, is not at all complicated. I want you to start focusing on eating high-quality, real foods, foods that spoil. This includes organic fresh vegetables, fruits, nuts and seeds, beans, unprocessed grains (preferably gluten-free), pasture-raised meats and eggs, wild-caught fish, and at least half your body weight in ounces of purified water daily. Before your mind jumps into a fury of food prison–like rules and regulations, I want to remind you that the list includes everything you would need to make a grass-fed burger over fresh greens, with a spicy side of sweet potato fries. Picture an adorable stack of silver-dollar pancakes (made from egg whites and oats) dripping with maple syrup, grass-fed butter, and a side of bacon. How about some homemade desserts naturally sweetened with dates, honey, and dark chocolate? Hold, please, I'm about to make some fish tacos with fresh guacamole, salsa, slaw, and cashew sour cream, and I won't feel like I'm giving up anything because it all tastes freaking orgasmic.

Here is a quick rundown of the things you want to minimize: processed foods (these come in a box or a bag), genetically modified foods (GMOs), flour, alcohol, soy, corn, artificial flavors and colors, trans fat and fried foods, sugar and high-fructose corn syrup, factory-farmed dairy, and (nonorganic) foods laden with pesticides, herbicides, and fungicides. Oh, and sugar, sugar, and more sugar! Did I mention any and all types of processed sugar? I could safely bet that you, my friend, at this very moment are addicted to sugar in some form or fashion (alcohol, bread, crackers, sweets, and pasta are all sugar, just dressed in different outfits). Sugar is a particular kind of evil that wreaks havoc on every body. Simply making sure that your food does not come from a package and is organic whenever possible will automatically protect you from eating anything on the above do-not-eat list. Then focus on minimizing all forms of processed sugar, and you'll be on the road to inner happiness! A simple rule of thumb is to keep your pantry bare and your fridge stocked.

Okay, okay, you read (or skimmed, yes, I saw that) the last paragraph, and you are feeling the sudden urge to give me the finger. It's cool, I get it, but truly I'm on your side, sugar-booger. I'm a foodie in the essence of my being. I have an inner fat kid who lives loud and proud! I know that a life without fries is not a life worth living, so I've created a loving boundary for myself that keeps me out of a food scarcity mentality.

I've been following this rule for years, throughout my weight loss and well into my weight maintenance. I eat whatever the hell I want twice a week. Two free meals. *Not cheat meals*, because I'm not cheating on anyone. I don't overeat, or binge on the most disgusting foods ever. I simply eat whatever sounds good, twice a week. That includes pizza, fries, bread, cheese, and of course pistachio coconut milk ice cream from my local Thai food joint. There's no food that I am *not allowed* to eat. I don't have to constantly check in with a running mental list of no-no's. When I started my quest for deeper and more permanent change, I created a vision for what I wanted regarding my health and physical appearance, and then I made loving boundaries that helped support my vision.

So the next time you find yourself wondering if you should eat this protein bar or that one, try the new fad food, or just say "F it" and get all those meals delivered in a box, you will know that the answer is to go with what spoils. Simply choose the fresh, real food option and win every time. This means a fresh cookie from the bakery wins out over a packaged one. It doesn't always have to be "healthy," but it should be real.

The next part takes a little more inner focus, and that is figuring out what ratio of foods make your particular body feel the best, look amazing, and poop like clockwork. In this step you will go on an inner quest. You will test the waters. And then you will become so in tune with your digestion that you will know without a doubt exactly what makes your body sing! Will the gurgles from your gut say, "I thrive on the paleo diet" or "I need to become vegan"? Well, obviously I can't tell you that just yet, but in either scenario, I promise you will find yourself eating mostly whole, real, unprocessed, and alive foods.

Finding Your Unique Medicine

Discovering the exact diet that works for you is easier than conventional wisdom makes it seem. Diet books try to convince you that you can't trust yourself and that therefore you need to follow the advice of someone who doesn't know the first thing about you. I know, it's cra-zay-zay. The truth is that we only have so many combinations to choose from, once we have cleaned most of the processed crap out of our diet. I know that cleaning the junky stuff out of our diet is easier said than done, but for this section, let's put emotion aside so you can at the very least learn what to do once you feel empowered enough to make those life-altering changes.

In the prior section, I discussed the simplicity of your eating foundation. To recap: Eat whole, unprocessed foods that rot and spoil. Eat lots of organic veggies, some fruits, grass-fed meats and eggs, wild fish, nuts and seeds, beans, gluten-free grains, and half your bodyweight in ounces of purified water. I drink reverse-osmosis water, but any filtered water is better than most tap water. Avoid processed sugar like the devil, and minimize caffeine, flour, alcohol, and processed junk. I know I sound like a bitch for adding the word *simplicity* to this concept because doing this day in and day out is anything but simple. I don't mean to invalidate the effort this takes, but the facts are the facts.

Finding your unique medicine refers to determining the ratio of these foods that works best for you. Do you thrive on a high-carbohydrate, moderate-protein, low-fat diet? Chances are if you do, you would feel great cutting out fatty meats and following the veganish diet principles. Do you feel best on a high-fat, moderate-protein, very low-carbohydrate diet? Then a ketogenic or paleo diet will create the results you have always dreamed of. Before you can answer these integral questions, you have to allow your body to call the shots, not the voice in your head.

Of the hundred-plus diet theories out there, the most logical explanation of biochemical individuality, the theory that different diets work for different people, was created by William Wolcott and Trish Fahey. Their book, *The Metabolic Typing Diet*, teaches that most people can put themselves into one of three different metabolic categories:

Protein types: Protein types (fast oxidizers) tend to be frequently hungry; crave fatty, salty foods; fail with low-calorie diets; and tend toward fatigue, anxiety, and nervousness. They are often lethargic or feel wired or on edge, with superficial energy while being tired underneath. These individuals do best on a low-carb, higher-fat, higher-protein protocol (think paleo).

Carbo types: Carbo types (slow oxidizers) have relatively weak appetites, problems with weight management, and type A personalities and are often dependent on caffeine. These individuals do best on a low-fat, lower-protein, higher-carb protocol (healthy vegetarians).

Mixed types: Mixed types are neither fast nor slow oxidizers. They have average appetites, cravings for sweets and starchy foods, and relatively little trouble with weight control. Mixed types have the most balanced diet, with equal ratios of protein, carbs, and fat.

Remember that this, like all other advice, is a guideline only. Ultimately it will be your individual body's response to dietary tweaks that will confirm whether or not you are on the right track. Once you bring more awareness to how your body responds to different ratios of food, you will likely notice a pattern forming. Try to drop your conditioned thoughts about food and receive guidance from your intuition (and digestive system!).

Too often I find people eating a certain way because a study or article told them it was the right way to eat. For example, they read an article about the paleo diet, and then all of a sudden lentils, a paleo no-no, give them digestive issues (whereas there was no physical response before they read the article). With all the information floating out there, it can prove very difficult to be neutral observer.

Our minds seek experiences that prove our thoughts to be true. I mean, who doesn't like to be right, amma right? The insane thing is that you will notice that you like to be right even when it causes you suffering. Say you had a partner in the past who cheated on you. Odds are that to protect yourself, your mind would create a story about how people are not to be trusted. You would likely put your focus on all the tales you heard about infidelity, and your mind would conveniently skip over any stories about couples experiencing loving, trustworthy relationships.

If this fascinates you, as it does me, I recommend David Allen's book *Getting Things Done*. In it he notes,

> Just like a computer, your brain has a search function — but it's even more phenomenal than a computer's. It seems to be programmed by what we focus on *and, more primarily, what we identify with.* It's the seat of what many people have referred to as the paradigms we maintain. We notice only what matches our internal belief systems and identified contexts. If you're an optometrist, for example, you'll tend to notice people wearing eyeglasses across a crowded room; if you're a building contractor, you may notice the room's physical details.

In other words, we see what we want to see.

If you have a friend who tried a high-fat, low-carb diet and gained five pounds, most likely you have doubts about this diet working for you. The same goes for the converse. If something worked for you in the past but isn't working for you now, it's hard not to repeat the old pattern, despite its lack of positive effect. Before you can talk to your body about its unique medicine, you must bring awareness to the stories you have about diets, what works and what doesn't, based on your past experiences. You must approach this with fresh eyes and a clean food slate.

Why You're Not Losing Weight

The human body is a complicated system, much more complicated than the theory of "calories in versus calories out." When the body is in balance, there is some truth to eating less and moving more, aka burning more calories than you consume. More often than not, however, we are stressed-out and hormonally out of balance. This makes it all too easy to pack on the pounds, despite our best diet and exercise efforts.

We live in a "cortisol culture," a culture that thrives on the idea that the harder you work, the more successful you become. Most people would rate themselves a 5 or more on a stress scale from 1 to 10. Even though we are sitting at our desks and not outside in loincloths running from our predators, we are still under a great deal of stress, putting our bodies in a chronic state of fight-or-flight. Our adrenal glands are pumping out cortisol and adrenaline, which eventually makes us feel burned-out, tired, and depressed. Since everything in our bodies is connected, if our stress hormones are out of balance, the odds are that our entire hormonal system is out of whack, thus taking a toll on our health as a whole. Ever hear the saying "stress will make you fat"? Our ability to burn stored fat as fuel is directly influenced by our state of hormonal balance, or lack thereof.

Shelly is a thirty-two-year-old single project manager for a tech firm in Austin. She works fifty-hour weeks, each day rushing home in traffic to let her poor dog out before he pees on the carpet. She is under constant stress from her job and feels like she could be fired at any minute. By the time the weekend rolls around, she is exhausted but feels pressure to go out and meet people. She wants to have a family but feels like time is not on her side. Every time she talks to her mother, she is reminded of how old she is when she hears, "Why haven't you signed up for online dating yet?" Shelly is also stressed about her body. She is fifteen pounds overweight from all the erratic food behaviors she's acquired from late nights at the office, with no time to cook. She drinks coffee to get going in the morning and wine to help her wind down at night. She goes to bed too late, her PMS is horrible, she gets sick a lot, her hair is thinning, and it feels like she gains weight much more easily than she can lose it. Because she constantly worries about her weight, Shelly has become an overexerciser, which only puts more stress on her body. This high-intensity exercise pumps out even more cortisol, which is blocking her ability to lose weight.

Shelly is a perfect example of the average hardworking woman. The stress she experiences is common in our culture and wouldn't raise much of an eyebrow in most people hearing of her daily grind. Her adrenals are fatigued, which in turn is affecting all her other hormonal glands. She has symptoms of underactive thyroid, estrogen dominance, weak immunity, and insulin resistance. These hormonal systems all work together. You can't put stress on one without putting stress on another. Soon enough, the entire system is off balance, causing Shelly to gain weight, which in turn makes her more stressed.

This never-ending cycle of stress, the body's response, and the reaction to the response can only be healed if we eliminate the root imbalance, which for Shelly is lack of self-care and a rotten belief system about never feeling enough. Shelly won't lose weight until she balances out her hormonal system, and that starts with lowering her stress. How do you know when your body is hormonally out of balance? You will experience any or all of the following: fatigue, trouble sleeping, food cravings, mood swings, severe PMS, and weak immunity.

Behavioral Patterns That Sabotage Weight Loss

If your stress levels are under a 5, on a scale from 1 to 10, and you don't resonate with the above list of symptoms for hormonal imbalance, the cause of your stubborn weight loss is most likely behavioral. There are always exceptions to the rules, but I have found that there are four behavioral patterns that sabotage our weight loss, and it's not hard to be stuck in at least three out of the four.

Overeating

Let's start with the most obvious, overeating. It's pretty hard these days to figure out the correct portion of food to eat, especially with dining out on colossal restaurant portions, eating on the run, and mindlessly snacking throughout the day. The practice of conscious eating, which we'll discuss further in chapter 6, will help you get in tune with your body's needs. The most general and effective rule of thumb is to eat, at one sitting, only what you can carry in your two hands.

Undereating

Most people are surprised by the second weight-loss roadblock, which is undereating. The science of this is pretty straightforward. The body needs a certain number of calories to sustain itself. Dropping below this number at first can cause weight loss. Stay there for too long, however, and your body will adjust your metabolic thermostat to function on a lower amount of caloric intake. Remember, your brain doesn't care if you look great in a bikini; its only job is to keep you alive. It will manipulate anything in the body to ensure your survival. Your thyroid produces a hormone called Free T3. This is the "flame" of your metabolism. Undereat for long periods, and T3 will lower the output of your metabolism. I know countless busy professionals who sacrifice their needs (like eating a solid lunch) to "get it all done" in the workplace.

They don't eat enough but don't feel hungry because they are jacked up on four cups of caffeine, which is an appetite suppressant. Eventually, the weekend rolls up, a friend comes into town, and they celebrate by increasing their calorie intake dramatically, and they do so on a slower metabolism. Poof, they gain weight quicker than a premenstrual woman at a Potato Chip Expo.

Wrong Ratio of Macronutrients

The next weight-dropping snafu is that you aren't eating the right ratio of protein, carbs, and fat for your unique medicine. I find that for most people, the exact ratio of protein, carbohydrates, and fat is the least of the roadblocks when all the other guidelines are in place. In fact, I think we drive ourselves crazy counting our calories and weighing our foods as a distraction from the deeper work we need to do to lose the weight. That being said, some of us will be much more sensitive to carbohydrates than others. When we eat carbohydrates (think beans, grains, potatoes, bread, pasta, crackers), they break down into sugar molecules. Sugar causes insulin to spike. Insulin is a hormone that removes the sugar from your blood and stores it as fat; you know, that "fuel for next time you need it" that you won't ever need because there is rarely a time with no meals or snacks.

The body has only two sources of fuel: glucose and stored fat. For people sensitive to carbohydrates, even eating what experts would consider a low-carb diet might be eating too many carbohydrates for the body to tap into its stored fat as a fuel source. If you suspect this might be an issue, try limiting your carbohydrates to unlimited green vegetables and one serving of berries, and hold off on the beans, legumes, grains, and starchy veggies until your body gives you feedback as to whether or not your insulin plays a factor here. If you start losing weight by limiting these carbohydrates, you can consider yourself sensitive to sugar.

Lack of Movement

The last, and one of the most likely, reasons that you may not be losing weight is that *you aren't getting enough exercise.* Unless you have a job that keeps you continually active, you will find that even a moderate exercise routine is not enough. Over the years I have acquired an affinity for working out. At times it's my favorite part of the day (did I just say that?!). I love getting sweaty, rocking out to music, and getting rid of any stuck negative energy. I typically exercise three to five times a week. I sound like an active Sporty Spice, don't I? Before I join the Spice Girls on tour, let's also consider that I sit while writing, coaching clients, and recording videos at least forty hours a week. So I'm active for three to five hours, and I sit on my butt for forty. Calculate the math for yourself right now. What's your ratio, and could this be your issue?

Despite having a consistent workout routine, I noticed a weight-loss plateau. I needed to take my fitness to the next level, but I didn't want to add any more squats or push-ups to my regimen. The thought of another workout class just didn't seem appealing. That's when I remembered the simple and overlooked art of walking.

I spent a month in London studying abroad. I ate out three meals a day and didn't pay much attention to my food choices. It would be safe to say that gaining a good ten pounds would have meant I lived it up. I did, however, walk everywhere and spent a few hours a day being active. When I came home and checked my weight, I hadn't gained an ounce. I am not one of those people. I gain weight on vacation, I gain weight eating carbs, I gain weight when I simply walk by a bakery and inhale. Instead of my normal routine of sitting for eight hours and moving for one, I was active for seven hours and sitting for two.

It's all about that activity. The only way to lose weight is to quit your job and move to Europe. I'm kidding. You may, however, need to add in many more walks during lunch, after dinner, and on the weekends. It's not always about increasing your workouts but increasing your overall movement.

If you try to manipulate these behaviors and still have no luck, I recommend that you see a holistic MD, a naturopath, a certified clinical nutritionist like myself, or someone you trust who can run lab tests and uncover the deeper issue for you. Whatever the case, do not lose hope. The body has a miraculous ability to heal itself, and no matter how long it has been imbalanced, it is always trying to restore itself to health. When you get healthy, your weight will stabilize as well.

Skimmer's Delight

- ✓ Being on a diet is not a bad thing. Everyone is on a diet. Make sure your emotions around your food protocol are positive and that you view any food rules as self-created loving boundaries that allow you to feel fantastic.
- ✓ You can transcend all diet dogma by making it a practice to eat foods that are unprocessed and alive — foods that rot and spoil make you feel alive!
- ✓ Heal your digestive issues so you can hear the body's feedback as to what is and isn't working.
- ✓ Finding your unique medicine is quite easy when you start listening to the true language of your body.
- ✓ Stress will cause hormonal imbalance, which makes it hard for you to lose weight. This should be addressed before you examine exercise and diet.

Make It Stick

1. Keep a food journal for the week, and see if you can connect your symptoms, emotions, and the consequences of those emotions to what you are eating.

2. Make a list of foods you consume that give you a stomachache or make you feel bloated, tired, and physically uncomfortable.
3. Make a list of foods that leave you feeling light, energetic, happy, and emotionally stabilized.
4. Create an intention statement based on this information. For example: "When I eat __________, I feel __________. However, when I choose to nourish myself with __________, I feel energetic, light, and happy. I commit to bringing a higher awareness to how food makes me feel."

chapter 6

CONSCIOUS EATING

silence the fat kid within

Between stimulus and response there is a space. In that space is our power to choose our response. In our response lies our growth and our freedom.
— Attributed to Viktor E. Frankl

Pasta doesn't make you fat. How much pasta you eat makes you fat.
— Giada De Laurentiis

Last night I received this email from a client: "I can't stop crying, and I just ate way too many spoonfuls of peanut butter… and then I'm pretty sure I pounded five stevia packets. I feel insane! I don't know how to fix this. The only cure I have ever had for my mood swings is food. What do I do???? I can*not* stick to this detox without some insight or discipline that I do not currently have. Please help!"

We've all been there, eating food to shift our emotions instead of addressing the emotion head-on by shifting our thoughts and taking back control of the voice in our head. You may never have found yourself eating pure stevia powder by the spoonful (may I suggest drinking maple syrup instead? — the mouth doesn't get as dry), but a cocktail, a box of crackers, or a serving of fries are fairly common self-medications for feeling shitty (which really means *thinking* shitty).

Why we engage in the behavior of eating is quite simple. There are only two reasons why we put food into our mouths.

1. We eat because we have a physical requirement to nourish the body with food.
2. We eat to change our emotional state to distract ourselves from what is causing discomfort.

It sounds simple, but since we can feel hundreds of different emotions, at times it feels like we eat for a hundred different reasons.

Every time you eat because you're bored, frustrated, happy, tired, heartsick, and so on, you are eating to shift your emotional state. If eating an entire box of gluten-free crackers with butter and jelly (I speak from others' experiences only; I've personally never done this while binge-watching old episodes of *Sex in the City*) causes me to shift my thinking about a specific area in my life, therefore leaving me with a deep peace and inner knowing, then I would be a huge proponent of eating your problems away. Who cares if you get fat? You will have no problems! Oh, wait, you will be fat and unhealthy, and that's a huge problem. There's also one small detail that we tend to overlook at the moment we are shoving our emotions deep down with food. This method just doesn't work! Not only does it not work, but it also creates an additional problem. Your first problem is whatever thought process was causing you to feel emotional discomfort; you can either change your thoughts or surrender and fully accept the present moment as it is. Your second problem is that you just ate a bunch of junk when you weren't hungry, and now you have to worry about your weight and your health, and whether the jeans you just bought will still fit you tomorrow. *Subconsciously, we eat to create a secondary problem when the primary issue is too overwhelming to deal with.*

I've been dealing with my weight and body image since I was in my teens. I may not like it, but trust me, this is an issue I'm used to dealing with. The unknown, on the other hand — that work situation, relationship stress, or family drama — I might not have the tools to work my way through that just yet. If I can distract myself with my feelings about weight and body image, then I don't have to deal with the real-life situation.

The term *conscious eating* gets thrown around a lot (much like the phrase *self-care*). Sure, you should eat slowly (just like you should meditate and take long baths), but have you honestly explored what conscious eating means to *you* as a daily practice? It's so much more than simply slowing down when you eat. It's cultivating a deeper presence, a respectful relationship between you, your mind, and the food you choose to consume. Conscious eating is a spiritual practice. It is not something to be mastered; you cannot just cross it off a to-do list. Just like any practice, with time it becomes more natural and more familiar, yet, as with most spiritual practices — forgiveness, patience, unconditional love, acceptance — you must set the intention every day to live in alignment with your practice, or it will humble the crap out of you.

Conscious Eating, Conscious Being

A kind of awareness beyond the thinking mind must occur for you to drive your food behaviors from your higher, more intuitive inner guide. To heighten this voice and make it easier to hear, you must practice awareness throughout the day, not just as you eat but as a constant state of being. I've never met anyone who was able to consciously eat and then mentally check out of the remainder of her day. This reminds me of an old saying: "The way we do anything is the way we do everything." To me it speaks to any behavior pattern causing some imbalance in my life. I can immediately ask myself, "How do I see this pattern show up in other areas?" The beauty of this practice is that it seeps into every aspect of your life. As you practice consciousness with food, you begin to practice consciousness of being, awareness of the present moment beyond the mind. This is precisely why it's impossible to separate permanent health from a deep spiritual path of self-development and exploration. Food is just a touchstone to show you where the work needs to be done for you to be healthier and happier as a whole.

This doesn't mean you have to be Buddha on a mountaintop to become a conscious eater. I go in and out of awareness all day long, just like everyone else. At times I feel incredibly present and unidentified with my mind's constant ramblings, and at other times I am staring into space, completely under the spell of whatever nonsense my mind is telling me, utterly unconscious to the present moment. The mark of your success is not how long you can stay in a fully aware and present state of being; it is how quickly you can recover to that place once you notice you're not there. As Eckhart Tolle teaches, "The word *enlightenment* conjures up the idea of some superhuman accomplishment, and the ego likes to keep it that way, but it is simply your natural state of felt oneness with Being.... Enlightenment consciously chosen means to relinquish your attachment to past and future and to make the Now the main focus of your life."

The Practice

I first learned to drive on Staten Island and Manhattan roads. I was one of those aggressive, cocky drivers you hated to share the road with. I was always in a rush, always speeding. I remember one of my ex-boyfriends (may he rest in peace. He's not dead, just dead to me) used to leave spare change in the side pocket of my door so when I would speed up and slow down the sound of the change rattling would annoy me. He would say, "If you can hear this change, you are going too damn fast." One day as I was speeding somewhere I'm sure was completely unimportant, my boyfriend pulled out his phone and read me a statistic that said that driving over the speed limit doesn't get you to your destination any more than a few minutes sooner. All that rush, all that stress, all that adrenaline, and all that risk for a measly five or so minutes?

Here's what I learned: that awful, frantic energy you expend on things throughout the day is not saving you any time! You could accomplish the same amount of work with an inner calm and grounded energy. Not only would you kick ass and take names, but you would also do it with much more clarity and ease. There is also so much more joy in the mundane, day-to-day tasks when you can slow down. You can be more cognizant of the beauty around you that you tend to miss when you are in a caffeinated, rushed-out-the-door frenzy. Now that you agree (I assume my story was convincing) that slowing down will help you make better decisions and increase your success in the long run, let's dive into the nitty-gritty of this practice. Get excited — it's guidelines time, baby!

Eat Only When You Are Physically Hungry

As you start your practice of conscious eating, first and foremost, you need to figure out why you just lunged for the fridge door handle. Is it because you are hungry, or is there an emotion that needs to be dealt with? Getting this answer can be as basic as asking yourself the question "Am I physically hungry?" If the answer is no, ask yourself a follow-up question: "What am I feeling right now that I'd like to shift?" In other words, what are you really "hungry" for? Do you need a quick break from that project you have been working on for the past few hours? Do you need comfort? Are you bored and needing something to do? You can use the tools I have given you to check in with your thoughts; they are the cause of what you are feeling. Can you reframe your thoughts to shift your emotion without the use of an external stimulus? That's the real deep spiritual work we are doing.

One of my oldest patterns was to reward myself for a job well done with sugary, glutenous, dairy-filled desserts. I'm certain this stems from my mother bringing my sister and me to Baskin-Robbins, you know, thirty-one flavors of chemicals, after we would get shots at the doctor or get an A on a test. My brain created the pattern "when you do well, you get a treat!" Woof woof.

Once I started the practice of conscious eating, I realized I was never hungry those times I grabbed my reward. I still wanted to reward myself; I just didn't think it was fair that my reward also created a consequence. I needed to find something that gave me that pat on the back, without it being detrimental to any aspect of my life. Instead of a cupcake (Congrats! You did so well, now you get to feel bloated), now I buy myself something small that doesn't break the bank. Or better yet, I'll treat myself to a gift that keeps on giving, such as a yoga class or a serene, introspective solo hike in the woods. Your patterns themselves may not be destructive; you may just need to change the reward to ensure that it is positive and consequence-free.

If you are craving a particular food in front of you but you aren't hungry, tell yourself that you can save it and eat it later without guilt as soon as you get the physical cue for hunger. If you are at a restaurant and get the signal that you need to stop eating, but you look down at your plate and the food looks so delicious that you start making up stories as to why you should keep eating, just interrupt your pattern by changing your physiology (get up and go to the bathroom, pick up your cell phone, walk outside to get some fresh air) and asking for a to-go box. Also, change your story by reminding yourself that this restaurant is not closing down and you can come back the very next day and eat this same meal again if you desire. Remove the preprogrammed mental scarcity story of the food going away or not being available again and replace it with a healthy dose of reality.

Many people mention not being able to truly tell if they are hungry. "Every time I ask myself if I'm hungry the answer I get is yes, but I can't tell if my stomach is answering or just my monkey mind." The ultimate truth is this: if you aren't sure whether or not you are hungry, you ain't hungry. When you are physically hungry, believe me, you will have no doubt. When you are hungry, your stomach feels empty, it starts twisting and pulsating, your blood sugar starts to drop, you begin to feel irritable, and you crave a legitimate meal, not a cookie.

Below is a detailed hunger scale for you to get accustomed to. The ideal scenario is that after a meal you feel satisfied with what you ate but you don't feel the food in your stomach. This means that your stomach didn't have to stretch beyond an appropriately sized portion for your body. That's how I know for sure I ate too much; I can feel the meal in my stomach, and it's uncomfortable. After a salad or a smoothie, for example, I feel renewed energy, but I don't feel anything in my stomach. This is your sweet spot!

The Hunger Scale	
0: Starving	Grumpy; headaches; dizziness
1: Hungry	Stomach growling
2: Could Eat	Not satisfied; hunger within an hour
3: Satisfied	Ideal state; can't feel food in stomach; lasts 2 to 3 hours
4: Full	Feel food in stomach
5: Too Full	Drowsy; unbuttoning pants; changing into sweats
6: Feel Sick	Too full to move; cursing food; stuffed

If you want to know for sure where you are on the hunger scale, always ask yourself the above questions with your eyes closed. Closing your eyes immediately shuts off external stimulus and puts you inside your body. Try this little experiment: Ask yourself right now if you are physically hungry. Once you get an answer, ask yourself the same question, but first close your eyes. See how easy it is to make discernments when you have nowhere to focus but within? I stumbled on this trick when I first started meditating. I would eat what I deemed an appropriate portion size, and then thirty minutes or so later I would sit to meditate. As soon as I closed my eyes, I would realize just how full I was from that meal. My hunger/fullness cues would heighten dramatically as soon as I sat in meditation. Now before and after I eat, I just shut my eyes, and I can feel my cues more intuitively.

Center Yourself before Each Meal or Snack

Take three slow, deep breaths and reflect on what type of emotions you are feeling and therefore bringing to the meal. Do you feel rushed, stressed, bored, or tired? How do you want to feel during and after this meal? Better yet, how you do want to feel the following day, the following week, and in the months to come? Clear out any funky residual energy from the past few hours by refocusing on how you want to feel about what you are eating, not about your experiences earlier in the day and your reaction to them.

Make a little space between you and your food so that as soon as you see or smell food, you're not diving into it face-first like Scrooge McDuck dives into a pile of money (you will only get this reference if you were a child of the '80s). Before you put food into your mouth, take a moment to think about the reward (pleasure) or consequence (pain) of this behavior. If what you are about to eat is not in alignment with what you want most, pivot your energy and thoughts so you can redirect and make a better choice.

Eat, and Do Nothing Else

Focus only on food when you are eating. Focus on things other than food when you are not eating. When the food is in front of you, put down your cell phone (I know, it's hard for me too), shut off the television, and just be with your food. Even if it's only for a short amount of time, you need to truly connect with what you are eating.

When you are finished eating, do absolutely anything but be around or focus on food. If you are home, get out of the kitchen. If you are at a restaurant, start asking your dinner partner some involved questions or walk outside. I always ask the waiter to take my plate as soon as I'm finished so I don't go back for those "but it's so delicious" last few bites that always put me over the edge.

Love Foods That Love You Back

I don't know what I ever did to piss off gluten and dairy, but they both hate me. They have made it very clear that I'm not in their little clique. Fine with me; I have enough alternatives, and I don't like to hang where I'm not wanted. Do I wish we could get along just for the sake of the occasional pizza? Of course, because I'm a lover, not a fighter. When I finally made my peace with food, I decided to write a code of conduct to outline the way I wanted to talk to myself and act around food.

One of my promises was to avoid constantly eating foods that cause physical discomfort to my body. Once in a while, I would deal with the consequences. In New York City? Eat a slice of pizza. In Italy? Have some gelato. Home on a Friday night and don't feel like cooking? Too bad, I better get something gluten- and dairy-free. You don't have to live 100 percent on or off anything, but decide to make a habit of loving food that loves you back. Practice honoring your body's communication system, and pay attention to what happens when you don't.

Eat as If You're a Professional Food Critic

Have you ever watched those food shows where the judges take a small bite of food and then talk about every aspect of its flavor? You can tell they genuinely love and celebrate the art of eating. We don't have to be at that level, but we could learn a thing or two from those judges on the Food Network. We need to slow down, plain and simple (see a theme forming here?). I used always to say I would overeat because I loved food so much, but the ugly truth was that I didn't love it *enough*. If you taste only one-tenth of your food's flavor, you are going to have to eat ten times as much to feel satisfied. You must notice the texture, smell, and temperature. Talk about the food, how it tastes, and what it feels like in your mouth. Use all your senses to heighten your eating experience. *More* joy from *less* food is the goal. No feeling of restriction. All pleasure. No consequence.

Halfway through Your Meal, Take a Breather

It's evident by now that to be a truly conscious eater you need to *slow the fuck down*. I can't tell you how many times I've opened a KIND bar and found that five seconds later the bar is gone, the wrapper is empty, and I'm checking my bra, convinced I must have dropped it into my cleavage because I didn't taste one stinkin' bite.

Slowing down when you eat (and when you do everything else in your life; remember, rushing only puts you five minutes ahead of schedule) will ensure that you make the time and space to think through your food decisions. Scientifically speaking, there is a substantial physiological benefit to this as well. In regards to your appetite, the body produces two hunger hormones. Ghrelin, produced in the lining of the stomach to increase hunger signals, tells us it's time to eat. Leptin, a hormone produced primarily by your fat cells, sends the message to your brain that you are full and that it's time to put the fork down. If you haven't already noticed, leptin takes its sweet time to get the message out. I like to think it has a lag time of about ten minutes. If you slow down your eating in general, you give the leptin enough time to get the signal to your brain. You will naturally feel full, and you won't need to force the feeling by finishing everything on your plate and feeling absolutely horrendous afterward. Halfway through the meal, set your fork down and place your attention on something else for five minutes. Self-soothe by telling yourself that if you are still hungry when you return to the food, you can continue eating. Use the abundance mantra: "There's always more."

You Bite It, You Write It

You can't manage what you don't measure. I'm not referring to measuring your food or counting calories, since that is the antithesis of healing your relationship with food! Plus, I'd rather do anything else in the world than look up how many calories are in a cup of strawberries. I'm talking about cultivating accountability and awareness by writing down the food you eat on a piece of paper or on the notes section in your cell phone. This allows you to more easily discover patterns and make connections as to *why* you are eating, *what* you are eating, and *when* you are eating. Added spiritual bonus: this is also a practice in nonjudgment as we take much-needed inventory so that we don't re-create destructive patterns.

Have a Morning and an Evening Self-Care Routine

Daily practices allow you to stay connected to your inner awareness and your intuitive eating guide. These rituals are vital to your long-term success! With the busyness that your day is likely to bring, anchoring yourself first thing in the morning and last thing at night will ensure you stay grounded and focused on what you truly want. In the next chapter we will dive into self-care: how to make it work for you and how to stop rolling your eyes when someone says you need more of it.

Skimmer's Delight

✓ **Eat only when you are physically hungry.** Ask yourself before you put anything into your mouth, "Am I physically hungry, or is this emotional hunger? What would really nourish me right now? What am I really hungry for?"

- ✓ **Center yourself before each meal or snack.** Before you put food into your mouth, take a moment to think about the reward and/or consequence of this behavior. If what you are about to eat is not in alignment with what you want most, pivot your energy and thoughts, and redirect to make a better choice.
- ✓ **Eat, and do nothing else.** Focus only on the food when you are eating. Focus on other things when you are not eating.
- ✓ **Love foods that love you back.** Avoid foods that cause physical discomfort to the body. Practice honoring your body's communication system, and pay attention to what happens when you don't.
- ✓ **Eat as if you're a professional food critic.** Slow down and enjoy every bite! If you taste only one-tenth of your food's flavor, you are going to have to eat ten times as much to feel satisfied.
- ✓ **Halfway through your meal, take a breather.** Set your fork down, and put your attention on something else for five minutes. Self-soothe by telling yourself that if you are still hungry when you return to the food, you can continue eating. Use the abundance mantra: "There's always more."
- ✓ **You bite it, you write it.** Writing down the food you eat allows you to see patterns and make connections to why you are eating what you're eating.
- ✓ **Have a morning and an evening self-care routine.** Daily practices allow you to stay anchored to your inner awareness and intuitive eating guide.

Make It Stick

1. Repetition is the practice of the experts. There is tremendous power in the lost art of handwriting. Every morning for seven days, rewrite the guidelines of conscious eating (bolded in the Skimmer's Delight above). As you write them, read them out loud to yourself.
2. What would change about your diet (and your body) if you loved only foods that loved you back?
3. Which of these guidelines is hardest for you, and why? What strategy will you use to ensure the daily practice of this particular guideline?

chapter 7

IT'S TIME TO DO YOU, BOO

Discipline equals freedom. — **Jocko Willink**

You've got to get up every morning with determination
if you're going to go to bed with satisfaction. — **George Lorimer**

I'm writing to you from a warm, sudsy bubble bath. The candles are lit, music is softly playing in the background, and I've got all the time in the world. No, I'm not. I'm lying. In fact, if one more self-care expert tells me to take a hot bath, I'm going to drown someone… right in that stinky bath I'm taking!

I understand why there is so much talk lately about redirecting our energy to self-care. Our culture is so obsessed with doing more to have more that we forget how to just *be* to feel fulfilled. We have become completely disconnected from our higher selves. We then have no choice but to make decisions based on what our minds are telling us, which we all know winds up being reactive and fear driven. Self-care allows us the space to ground and connect to our deeper purpose, our more conscious selves. I know you yearn to have that feeling of inner connectedness and a deep, peaceful knowing without having to take a bubble bath all the time. Never fear; I will teach you how to incorporate daily self-care into your already-too-busy life.

If you want to lose weight permanently, you have got to take care of yourself and connect to the wise and all-knowing voice that lies underneath the daily chaos. How about you and I make a deal? I'll help you solidify your self-care rituals if you commit to thirty days of a twice-daily self-care check-in. Let's witness what happens along your health journey. My promise to you is that I will never ask you to take a bath, although if you finally want to use all those bath beads you've been collecting since the '90s, then light some candles, throw on some Boyz II Men, and do your thang. You in? Then read on, you badass self-care warrior.

The Nightmare We Are Living

Jackie wakes up to her third alarm, and within the first ten minutes of being awake, she picks up her phone to check her email. (I'm going to call this person Jackie, but I'm actually talking about you. We also know "Jackie" is checking her phone while she's on the toilet, but we will keep this scenario classy and leave her some dignity.) She immediately feels stressed as she begins to make a list of all the things she has to accomplish at work. She rushes to get ready, already late because she pressed the snooze button one too many times. She has no time for breakfast, so she grabs a coffee on the way into the office. She considers it a victory that she didn't grab the morning pastry, and her story is "nothing is better than something bad."

Her day is chaotic. It's a back-and-forth between meetings, answering emails, and making personal lists, and honestly, her weekends don't look much different, with the nonstop errands and social commitments. She eats lunch at her desk while she works, thinking it's better to go straight through and get out early. On the way home, she checks her phone at every red light, oblivious to the world around her.

She spends the rest of the night on the couch watching TV and eating popcorn, counting down the minutes until it's Saturday and she can sleep in.

There are many versions of this story. Perhaps you are managing to fit in four to five days a week of exercise, but you still rush through the process, never fully present in the moment and always planning the hour ahead of you. Maybe you settle in from the day, and instead of eating popcorn in front of the boob tube you finish off a bottle of wine or a pint of ice cream. Perhaps you are spearheading an entire family unit. You are super mom, super organizer, and super wife, with an unending list of to-do's. We all have lived some iteration of this day, which, regardless of the details, is a day in which you feel disconnected, distracted, and completely identified with the voice in your head. There's no self-care, and no awareness, and it's going to lead you down the rabbit hole of out-of-control emotions, outbursts, overwhelm, and poor eating decisions.

It's Time to Do You, Boo

We have already laid the groundwork for your permanent change. You now know that true change starts with the mind. You have begun to rewrite your stories and to examine core beliefs so that you can attach pleasure to what will bring you the most long-term happiness and success. You are reframing the word *stress* and starting to feel more empowered and in control of your emotions and reactions. It's now time to do *you.*

I consider five top nonnegotiables when it comes to self-care: (1) sleep, (2) cooking, (3) exercise, (4) meditation, and (5) silence. There's no way around it; these just gotta get done. When you incorporate these fantastic five into your life, you will find that your health will start to improve dramatically, without your even having to focus on your weight. Each of these self-care pillars takes hard work, and time management, but you are beyond worth the effort! The power you have lies within the story you create around these self-care principles. These can't be painful for you to incorporate, or else you won't stay consistent. You must work your language and your focus to make self-care feel pleasurable. It starts with believing that you are worth it, that doing these things will create the life you desire, and that there is time to get it all done.

Sleeping (and Fat-Burning) Beauty

I've done some weird shit to lose weight. I've gone to back-to-back workout classes, tried fad diets, and drank three disgusting premade smoothies a day in place of meals. There have been times when if you told me that sticking a hose up my butt could help me lose weight, I would have done it (okay, I've done that too and wound up pooping on the rug in the waiting room, but that's a different story for a different time). I bet that at some point you have fallen into this category of desperation. Maybe it's not desperation, but a strong will, a burning desire, and a loose mental screw. Before you go booking your colonic, know that I got your backside. I'm going to share the ultimate secret. I happen to know of something that helps you lose weight while you lay completely still, no push-ups required. Sounds like the best deal ever, so why are you staying up so late binge-watching episodes of a show you have seen twenty times? Go to sleep!

If you are trying to lose weight, balance your hormones, or bring sanity back into your life, the amount of *zzz*'s you get might be just as important as what you eat and how much you exercise. It's been proven that a sleepy brain craves high-carb junk and lacks impulse control. Lack of adequate sleep messes with your brain chemistry, and low serotonin causes us to crave sugar. Hormonal imbalances and physical injuries to the body don't get a chance to heal fully, and your frazzled nerves and weak adrenal glands start a fresh new day on 50 percent battery. It won't be long before the thyroid starts to poop out from too many late nights and stressful days. If the physiology of this doesn't have you heading straight for that pillow, then take a moment to visualize how different your life would be if you didn't wake up at the last possible minute. You could create a morning routine that allowed you to upgrade your entire life. For all these reasons, getting an average of eight hours of sleep a night, between 10 PM and 6 AM, is self-care nonnegotiable numero uno.

Go to Bed as If You're Getting Paid, and Wake Up as If It's Your First Day on Vacation

No adult argues the pleasure of getting a deep night's sleep in a warm, cozy bed. It's the pain of going to sleep early and waking up early that's the problem. Here are my two favorite tools to help me get my butt into bed on time so I can wake up early and start the day with intention.

Mel Robbins, a well-known author and speaker, and the creator of the five-second rule, teaches that there is only one rule for getting what you want. That one rule is: you are never going to feel like it. If you only did the things you don't feel like doing, you would have everything you've ever wanted, but you don't because you give the mind enough time to talk you out of it. From the moment you have the idea to do something, you have only five seconds to take action, or else it's gone. Your brain will swoop in so fast to tell you all the reasons why you don't feel like it, and then before you know it you have hit snooze, rolled over, and given a giant middle finger to your productivity that day. What you need to do is simple. As you set your alarm each night, think about all the amazing things you will do with the extra time in the morning. Visualize waking up refreshed and popping out of bed as if it's the first day of your beach vacation. When the alarm goes off in the morning, immediately start counting down from five, four, three, two, one...and then open your eyes, place your feet on the ground, and think the words *thank you.* Wake up in a state of gratitude for the adventure you are about to have.

The day is over, you have kicked ass, and now you are relaxing on the couch watching TV and having some "you" time. It's hard to rip yourself away, and going to sleep feels like you are cutting your self-care time short. The second you think about going to sleep, count down from five, four, three, two, one and shut off the TV, put down the book or your phone, and go to bed as if you are getting paid for every hour of that healing shut-eye. By changing this habit and getting more consistent sleep, you are welcoming opportunity and abundance into your life in a way you never could before.

Since you are such a badass thought-shifting expert by now, you can recognize a rotten behavior from miles away. If you are having trouble waking up in the morning despite all these tools, it's the disempowering story you tell yourself that requires your attention and your rewrite. What is the very first thing you said to yourself when you woke up this morning? I'll be honest, my first thoughts this morning were, "Ugh! I could sleep for four more hours." I immediately caught that nasty thought before my hand hit the snooze button and I reframed right away to, "The day is here, and I am grateful to be alive. There are people my age in a hospital bed right now, and in honor of them I am going to wake up and move my body." What would be the best possible mantra for you when your eyes open and you greet the day?

A note to parents: I understand you are coping with interrupted sleep and that some things are just not in your control. That being said, you know those nights where you fall asleep at 8 PM while reading books and snuggling with your kiddos? Well, now this is your bedtime too! As alluring as cleaning up the kitchen, packing the school lunches, and prepping for the next day may be, getting shut-eye and waking up earlier to accomplish what you skipped the night before will do wonders for your hormones.

Never Trust a Skinny Cook

Growing up, I had a close friend whose mother was Italian. Her mother was a heavyset woman with beautiful olive skin and long, dark, curly hair. Sure, I enjoyed playing with Nicole, but my favorite part of going to her house was the chance to stay for dinner. The kitchen always smelled like tomato sauce and basil. We ate foods like homemade focaccia, meatballs with ricotta, lasagna, and fresh gnocchi with pesto. Her mom always wore an apron that said "Never trust a skinny cook." I found it funny at the time because my mom was naturally thin and a marginal cook at best (sorry, Mom, I love you, but creamed spinach in the microwave was not your finest moment). Anyhoo, it was obvious to third-grade me that Nicole's mom was the Emeril Lagasse of all moms. And furthermore, the apron was obviously wise beyond its sauce-stained years.

Still, I have to ask myself, is there some real truth to this slogan? I would say never trust a cook (skinny or not) who is making food for the sole purpose of flavor and not taking health into account! Unfortunately, that statement describes the food prepared at 99 percent of all restaurants. Have you ever eaten something at a restaurant that you also make at home and said to yourself, "Wow, it never tastes like this when I make it"? That's because it's probably flash-fried, sopping with oil, or coated in GMO corn.

I recently went to a hip and trendy new Asian place that sources grass-fed beef for their dishes, and they openly admitted to using MSG to make their "flavors pop." MSG?! What century is this, people? The fact is, you just never know what's in your food unless you cook it yourself. I call this phenomenon the consumption of "invisible foods" because you can't see the four hundred extra calories that came along with those "crispy" Brussels sprouts. Let's not fool ourselves; those sprouts are just French fries in frilly green dresses.

Not too long ago I took an old friend, who was on a strict candida diet and had to avoid any and all sugar, out to dinner. Being the health nut that I am, I was happy to show off my go-to healthy eatery and took her to a local Thai food joint that uses farmers' market veggies and pasture-raised meats. When she told the waitress she couldn't eat any sugar whatsoever, the waitress told us she would double-check with the chef and then let us know what was safe. She came back with a hesitant look on her face and said, "Actually, the chef said everything has sugar in it except for the salad." My friend looked at me as if to say, "Why the $%#! did you take me here?" and so under pressure, I started pushing back. "What about the coconut soup? The curry? The veggie stir-fry?" Yep, everything has sugar. Sugar, sugar everywhere, and not a drop to drink (or gallons to drink if you're still on the soda train).

Listen, I'm not telling you never to eat out again; I am simply making it clear that you cannot trust strangers with your health. You cannot put your health in the hands of the chefs at a restaurant whose only goal is for you to come back in order to drive food sales. For this reason, self-care nonnegotiable number two is to *cook your own food the majority of the time.*

The strategy for this is clear-cut. You have to plan a week's worth of dinners before the week begins. I don't care if you have a super nerdy spreadsheet computer document, if you use a shared app with household members, or if you kick it old-school with a whiteboard that you keep in your kitchen. Any method that fits your lifestyle will do the trick; you just need to write down a plan before you make your weekly grocery list. To make this strategy your own, you must decide the following:

1. **How many times are you willing to eat out per week?** I want you to keep this number at four or under. This includes any meal you eat out, so watch those sneaky lunches! Write this into your weekly plan by using a question mark in place of where you would write down your home-cooked meal. Once you figure out where you are eating, take a look at the menu beforehand and decide what the best option will be for you. Then write that exact meal in your meal plan before you head to the restaurant. This will greatly increase the likelihood of your sticking to the choice you made when you had clarity about how you wanted to feel

after the meal. Try to avoid choosing your meal when you are starving, tired, and smelling everyone else's food. For some sick reason, the folks at the table next to me always order the three unhealthiest dishes on the menu. Now I ask you, am I gonna order the salad on a whim once I get a whiff of those duck-fat-infused fries? Just, no.

2. **How many times are you willing to eat leftovers?** I only like to eat leftovers once. After that, I don't enjoy my food, which makes me crave all sorts of crap. Every time I make a dish, I make myself two servings' worth. To make my weekday easy, I almost always eat for lunch the meal I had for dinner the night before. At the time you plate your dinner, also put your lunch portion in a glass container for the next day.
3. **What days are best for you to cook, taking into account your other commitments?** If you can cook every night and prefer to eat fresh, then that's awesome! Once I retire, I will make a fresh meal every night. For this period in my life, batch-cooking works best for me, and I assume it will also work best for you. Take into account your exercise plan, family obligations, social plans, and so forth and come up with the best days for committing an hour or so to the kitchen. When I batch-cook, I come up with two meals to cook at once. One meal is usually a Crock-Pot dish, an easy throw-everything-on-the-grill type of meal, or a one-pot casserole that I throw in the oven and fuhgeddaboudit. That way, while it's cooking, I can focus on making a slightly more labor-intensive meal (any meal that requires a homemade dressing or sauce, requiring an extra step or two). Because I want to start the week focused and strong, I batch-cook on Sunday, when I have plenty of time to be in the kitchen. By Wednesday I need to do it again, and by Friday, my fridge is empty and

I usually go out to eat (or to my mom's...hey, Ma, not complaining about your cooking now, am I?). Saturday is my food-shopping day, and then on Sunday, I batch-cook all over again.

I know this sounds rigid, but I promise you this self-care nonnegotiable needs to be set in stone for you to be successful. Go to the grocery store on the same day (almost) every week. Prep and cook on the same days to turn this routine into a self-loving ritual. As always, make room to zig and zag every now and then. If you have an unexpected dinner guest, throw your leftovers into the freezer for a time when you don't feel like cooking. Don't be afraid to throw away food if your plan didn't go as you'd hoped. You will try to avoid wasting food at all costs, but don't stress about this as you get into the groove.

Going away on vacation for a week? Before you leave, make your weekly plan for when you get home. When you get back into town, head right to the store with your already-planned-out list, and start the week back in full-on self-care mode. If this means remembering to put your list in your car so you can head straight to the store from the airport, then yes, I have officially turned you into an anal-retentive food shopper, woohoo! More important, I promise that you will feel amazing once you get home, unpack, shower, and realize that you already have a fridge full of delicious, fresh food. Too often people eat more destructively the weeks *after* they get home from vacation than they did on the vacation itself. They return home, jumping back into work and life, and it takes them three weeks to get back in the groove, when the vacation was only one week long.

If you are making a Crock-Pot recipe, think about making a few portions to freeze for future meals or for unexpected guests. If you have a partner who is a bottomless pit, like my husband, having an extra meal on hand can help keep the hangries away and ease the overall flow of your week. If you have a busy week ahead, make sure to keep the meals simple but delicious. Don't worry about being perfect; using little shortcuts when you make meals is still so much better than eating out. If you plan a meal that calls for walnut pesto but you know by the end of the week you won't be able to tell your ass from your elbow, good god, please buy premade pesto and throw some walnuts on top of your dish.

Once you have your three to five meals planned out, make a grocery list from the selected meals. I used to go to the grocery store without a list and pick up the same five pieces of produce, some random meat, and so on. Then I would get home and not want to make or eat anything that I bought. Every evening, the task of cooking dinner began with staring into the abyss of random ingredients that was my fridge. I wound up making seventeen hundred different veggie stir-fries with random ground meats thrown on top of them. Inevitably, I would then eat any sweet thing I could find in my house in a futile attempt to find satisfaction after every one of those oh-so-health-conscious meals.

4. **How will you come up with your meal ideas?** This can be the most dreaded part of the entire process if you aren't prepared. Since I like to cook heavy veggie meals free of dairy, gluten, and sugar, I find recipes on vegan blogs and in cookbooks that I can add meat to. I then do the same thing with paleo recipes and add beans or gluten-free grains, if I'm feeling fancy. Go to a used bookstore and buy some amazing cookbooks. Go home and read them cover to cover, earmarking any recipes you will make in the future, so you

aren't thumbing through the entire book every weekend. Think of it as creating cookbook CliffsNotes. I'm super jazzed if I get two or three solid recipes from one cookbook into regular rotation. Create a folder on your computer (I have a Mac, so I used the bookmarks tab and created a designated recipe folder) and start following online blogs, such as mine (shameless plug)! There are so many free resources online for healthy, delicious meal ideas. Bookmark the recipes you like so you can easily go back to your favorites. There are also endless apps that will customize a meal plan and grocery list for you.

5. **How are you going to attach pleasure to this?** We know this is the most important piece of the puzzle, since this mind work is the foundation of all your future batch-cooking behaviors. Whether or not you become an avid cook will depend on the pain and pleasure you associate with this self-care principle. I want you to take the most painful part of the process and reframe it to attach pleasure. If you hate parking at the grocery store, just take the farthest spot automatically, and as you walk up to the store, take that two minutes to think about everything you are grateful for. If it's the chopping and prepping that annoys you to no end, put on music or play a movie on your computer. If it's cleaning the dishes you hate (I'm in this category), count this time as a meditation. Can you be completely present and intentional about cleaning every dish? Time yourself, or listen to a podcast or an audiobook, and when you are done, make sure to stand back, look at your beautifully clean kitchen and the nourishing food in your fridge, take a deep breath, and know you are on top of your game.

Just a reminder, if attaching pleasure just isn't working, then do the opposite. Attach massive amounts of pain to not doing it. If you don't cook, you will waste tons of money eating crappy food that is going to make you fat and sick. I don't attach pleasure to flossing my teeth every night, but there's more pain in yellow, rotting teeth and swollen gums than there is in flossing. Choose the story that works best for you.

Free Drugs

I started exercising in high school because I wanted to lose weight. In no way did I enjoy it, but even then I knew that I was going to have to move and be active if I wanted to feel good about myself. A few months in, something amazing happened. Working out became enjoyable. I started feeling stronger, and my workout began to give me a high that lasted all day. It helped with my anxiety, it improved my sleep quality, it improved my digestion, and I felt more energetic as a whole. Exercise was like free party drugs! If you like to party, then subscribe to self-care nonnegotiable number three.

Along with the feel-good endorphins that exercise provides, it also provides you with the calorie burn you need to lose weight and keep it off. It's impossible to lose weight using diet alone. Sure, you could eat a lot less and lose weight by cutting calories, but that method will come back to bite you in the ass. Every study showing that diets don't work long-term is referencing this physiological truth. Your body will get used to the lower intake, and your thyroid will lower your rate of metabolism to keep the body functioning on less nutrition. Your best option is to eat lots of healthy food and move your body accordingly. I could go on and on about the benefits of exercise, but you know that it's a must for a healthy mind, a lean body, and robust aging. Instead of boring you with endless facts and studies, I'd like us to get right down to business and set up the structure of your exercise routine.

Despite the contradictory recommendations on the cover of every fitness magazine, it doesn't matter, at the end of the day, what exercise you choose to do. Could you tailor exercise in a painstaking way to suit your exact needs? Yes, and like most other things, you will drive yourself crazy in the process. The most important factor in your exercise routine is not whether you lift weights, do cardio, or go to Pilates. The single most important factor predicting the success of your exercise routine is that you do it consistently, week after week, month after month, year after year. Yes, you should do different exercises, switch up your routine, and push yourself to improve, but honestly, we get so caught up in the details that we forget it doesn't matter as much as simply showing up to do it! Depending on where you are starting (couch potato or avid overexerciser who needs to rest more), I suggest you try a well-rounded routine. This includes some heavier, shorter-duration exercise such as thirty minutes of jogging, speed walking, spin class, or resistance training, as well as some longer, less intense movement like an hour-long yoga class, a long hike or walk, Pilates, or slow swimming. If you exercise too much, your mantra needs to be to do less. If you don't move enough, get an accountability partner to help you increase consistency. Or get a trainer, and pay someone to watch as you breathe heavily and sweat from all kinds of unattractive places.

Whatever you decide to do, make sure it's something you enjoy, attaching as much pleasure to the exercise as you can. Aim to move five to six days a week, leaving a day or two to be completely lazy. Get a massage, use a foam roller, and take care of your body so that it takes care of you for a long time to come.

The Calm Behind the Neuroses

The mind is so busy at all times, it feels like an anxious, judgmental hamster running on one of those wheels. The mind and emotions are so interconnected that if our minds are always going, our bodies are always responding. This sucks precious energy that we can't afford to waste. The constant stream of thought makes it hard to hear that intuitive voice we rely on to make the most loving and wisest health choices throughout the day. This makes meditation and silence self-care nonnegotiables four and five. In other words, you gotta know when to shut it down and just shut up.

The most important lesson I learned while practicing meditation was that the intention of meditation is not to shut "off" the mind. Try right now to shut off the mind. I'll give you a million dollars to not think for the next ten minutes. Stopping the mind from thought is like trying to stop a moving train by standing in front of it with your hands out. Instead, the purpose of meditation is to quiet the mind, to allow thoughts to move effortlessly through you like a stream of water, not attaching to any one thought. Once I understood the distinction between absence of thought and not attaching to thought, my meditations became much more enjoyable.

There are so many different ways to nourish your meditation practice, depending on where you are on the journey. If you are a beginner, instead of starting at home or doing it yourself using an app, I suggest you find a local meditation center or teacher and experience the way meditation was always traditionally taught, directly from teacher to student. This will put you light-years ahead on your path to becoming a deep and consistent meditator. If you don't live in a location that has these resources (which I will say these days is rare), check out Transcendental Meditation (tm.org) or Neelakantha Meditation (bluethroatyoga.com).

Another way to meditate is to have periods of silence when you can truly go within and redirect that outward energy toward inward healing and reflection. I always suggest doing this in nature, if possible, as it intensifies the experience. How much silence you need will be up to you and your individual personality. If you tend to be a social butterfly, live with a roommate, or have a very social job, I suggest you do this more often than someone who regularly spends a lot of time alone. For me, once a week, I need to shut off my cell phone, go outside for a hike or at the very least put my bare feet in the grass, and go a few hours without speaking to anyone. Regardless of the specifics, as with all five self-care nonnegotiables, you need to preplan and make room for this in your weekly schedule. What is a "should" almost never happens, but what you consider a "must" always gets done. For me, if it ain't written down in a calendar, it ain't happenin'.

Resources vs. Resourcefulness

I know all these self-care nonnegotiables sound fantastic in theory. You can just picture how relaxed, healthy, and toned you would be if you were the type of person who had "that kind of time." I can just hear your story: "If I didn't have __________ [insert your reason for why your time is limited: kids, a useless husband, a demanding job, a sick parent, a social life], then I would be able to spend three hours every day cooking, meditating, exercising, and walking in nature." If your story isn't about time, then it's most likely about your other precious resource: money. "If only I had the money to spend on boutique fitness, a chef, and a nanny." Honey, I hear ya. But I'm no Oprah, either.

I had stories of my own when it came to my self-care. They were the same ones we just mentioned, only probably a little more dramatic sounding because in case you haven't noticed, I have a flair for the dramatic. If you've never met someone who could turn self-care into stress, well then, nice to meet you. I couldn't just read a blog; I needed to cook, meditate, exercise, dry-brush my body, oil-pull, do yoga, roll out the bottom of my feet, exfoliate my face, get to sleep on time, make my chiropractor and massage appointments, sit in my infrared sauna that didn't exist, read for pleasure but also to grow my mind, and the list went on. Finally, I got a grip on my self-care using these guiding principles.

First, you cannot break down your self-care rituals into a long list of these little to-do's. You have to shift your frame of mind (are you sick of my saying that yet? Because we still have a few more chapters to go) and think of your self-care as an attitude, an approach to life. You don't have to do all these things daily; no one is going to prioritize that much time. Instead, you need to make a list of your top five nonnegotiables and start fitting them into your calendar. Some of these principles only need to occur for you once or twice a week, and others every day. Put a recurring appointment on your calendar for a silent hike or a cell-phone-free day. Solidify your exercise and batch-cooking routine and add that to your calendar as well. For the daily nonnegotiables, make your own unique twice-daily ritual.

Second, you have to understand the difference between your resources (time, money, and other people) and your resourcefulness. No matter how rich or famous you are, you have only three resources available. You may have more of one resource than another (I find that the more money someone makes, the less time she typically has), but it only comes down to these three. On the other hand, your resourcefulness, meaning how you use what you have, is limitless. If you don't have a lot of money, think of something you can trade with another person to get what you need.

I had a client who desperately wanted to get her child into daycare at a Montessori school. She was complaining to me about how stressed-out she was because she couldn't afford the school but wanted to give her daughter the best education and care she possibly could. At the time she was working in human resources at a local public school. I suggested that she inquire about any job openings at Montessori so that her child could go to school for free, and the next time I saw her she had switched jobs, and with the tuition covered, she was making the same money! She traded her time resource to get what she most needed. When I first started my business, I couldn't afford to hire employees, so I posted internship opportunities at the local college. I knew students would need the internship for credit, and they could help me in my business. I traded my knowledge for someone else's time. I have a high-powered client who has the money to spend on her health but not the time. She's on a plane twice a week. For this unusual schedule, we put together an entire self-care routine she can do while she's on the plane, ensuring that she makes the most of her valuable resource: time. Look at the state of your resources. Do you have some money to delegate to your self-care? Or is it time you have more of? Start to think creatively about this, and you will exponentially increase your ability to stay consistent.

Set Up Your Twice-Daily Rituals

Your twice-daily ritual shouldn't take you more than five to twenty-five minutes in the morning and at night. Whatever time you allow for this, the more important piece is that it becomes a ritual, something that you are pulled toward with tremendous discipline. If movement is what feels best first thing in the morning, perhaps your morning ritual looks like ten minutes of yoga, five minutes of meditation, and three minutes of intention setting. If you are dedicated to a longer meditation practice, adjust your time accordingly. I suggest having a spot in your room or home that you go to each morning to help with repetition.

My morning ritual is as follows: I wake up, turn on my lavender essential oil lamp, and meditate for twenty minutes. I have two alarms set three minutes apart so that after my meditation is complete, I sit in gratitude for three minutes, and the final three minutes I visualize myself going through my day. I picture the way I want to eat and the choices I want to make, and I imagine myself going through the day with a calm inner sense of being. After the final bell, I get up, do some light stretching, and start my day. My evening ritual is to do some light stretching and journaling about the day. I put on soft music and take deep, slow breaths as I wash away any stickiness from the day. This evening ritual only takes me five to ten minutes.

I promise you that by taking the time to connect with yourself each day, you are exponentially strengthening your intuitive voice. This voice reassures you with your new core beliefs. This is the same voice that gives you the best advice on what and when to eat and how to eat it. This voice pulls you out of judgment, comparison, and fear. You need this voice to lead a happy life, and you need self-care to hear this voice. Self-care is ultimately what allows you to lose weight and keep it off. Without it, all you have is a diet.

Skimmer's Delight

- ✓ Self-care is the absolute most important aspect of permanent change.
- ✓ The five nonnegotiables of weight loss, health, and vitality are sleep, cooking, exercise, meditation, and silence.
- ✓ Morning and evening daily rituals will help keep you grounded and clear on what you want most.
- ✓ Saying you don't have time is the same as saying you don't want to make time. We make time for the things we value.
- ✓ You are never going to feel like doing the things you need to do. Use the five-second rule to help you take massive action!
- ✓ You will never feel like you have enough resources — but how *resourceful* you are with what you've got will make all the difference.

Make It Stick

1. Create an empowering wake-up statement that you repeat every morning as soon as your eyes open. Some examples:
    - It's going to be a great day today!
    - This day is a gift, and I'm going to squeeze every moment out of it!
    - I love life; now it's time to get up and live it!
2. Take some time to create a strategy for your five self-care nonnegotiables. First, make a list of items you will need and people you can call on to include in your journey or to help you stay accountable. Last, schedule all these self-care behaviors and set alarms to trigger you into engaging in new patterns.

PART THREE

find your true self

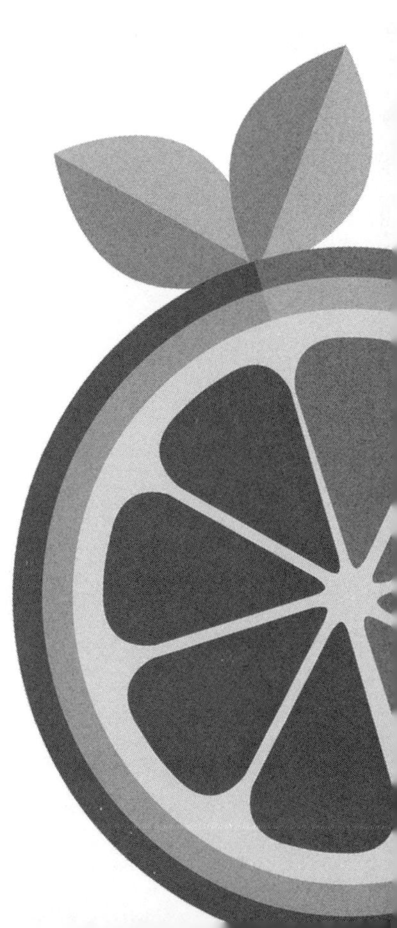

chapter 8

YOUR BODY IS A WONDERLAND

Each individual woman's body demands to be accepted on its own terms.
— Gloria Steinem

Everybody has a part of her body that she doesn't like, but I've stopped complaining about mine because I don't want to critique nature's handiwork.... My job is simply to allow the light to shine out of the masterpiece. **— Alfre Woodard**

I will never forget the time when my sister's (then) boyfriend had come to visit for the weekend, ruining all my sister/roommate bonding plans, as usual. Only this time, he had a surprise in store. He brought his little brother along with him for a visit. He was so handsome in that just-turned-nineteen kinda way. Unfortunately, he was also tall, muscled out from a teenage passion for gymnastics, *and* a freckled redhead, so naturally, I decided to devour him whole. After finishing our first morning sexathon, I was tidying up the clothes strewn about the room when he pointed to my thigh and said, "By the way, what is that?" I was in such a postcoital stupor that at first the question didn't register. "What is what?" I asked, unknowingly spinning myself deeper and deeper into the impending shame spiral. "Those dents in your thighs. Are they scars, or what?" As soon as I heard the words *dents in your thighs*, my stomach dropped. My mind began to race, and I tried to think of the best possible answer that would allow me to hold on to some shred of dignity. I wanted to scream, "That's just my thigh, you fool! It's called cellulite, and it is what they artfully airbrush off all the chicks in your porno mags. Haven't you ever seen a real woman before? Dimples show up on more than just my smile, asshole!" But if I remember correctly, my answer was: "Oh, I don't know."

It was one of the most embarrassing moments of my life. Here I was, prancing around like an uninhibited sex goddess, only to be completely deflated after one innocent little question. The shame I felt about suddenly no longer seeming perfect in his eyes was simply a mirror for how I truly felt about myself. The poor guy wasn't trying to be mean. The reality is that he probably had never seen a curvy-bodied, real-life naked woman before. His only fault was not yet knowing the things you don't say to a woman. How could he have possibly known that he was pointing out my most-hated body part?

On the surface, I brushed it off and then got him out of my apartment as soon as possible. It wasn't that freckled teenager I could no longer face; it was the shame I carried with me for so many years about this seemingly huge imperfection. I wished at that moment that I was confident enough to explain that even though I was in the best shape of my life, my thighs had cellulite... and that it was perfectly okay (and so are my chin hairs, random varicose veins, and the one nipple that I swear is bigger than the other).

I obviously had some work to do around accepting my body and all its imperfections. Once I understood that it wasn't my body but my mind that was the problem, I realized the work I had to do was not in the gym but in my head. I didn't need to swing in the opposite direction and brainwash myself to believe that these were the most beautiful parts of my body. I just changed my story to neutralize my emotion around it. Cellulite might not be the most attractive part of me, but that's okay because there are so many other great things for me to focus on, both inside and out. We have to accept our bodies for what they look like right now, if we ever hope to feel motivated to change.

Often we are unwilling to accept ourselves out of fear that acceptance will kill our motivation. If we accept where we are, then why should we change it? We worry that accepting our bodies will leave us sucked into the couch. However, the opposite is true. Once we accept and truly make peace with exactly where we are on our journey, we can start working with ourselves from a place of love, respect, and genuine connection with our true selves.

True Change Happens by Love, Not Force

Body image and food chaos are directly related. The worse we feel about ourselves, the more we feel that punishment is the only way to produce change. We force a diet or workout regimen without examining where this compulsion is coming from. The regimen never sticks long-term, and that's a fact. I would eat so poorly for a period of time that my only window to salvation was to punish myself with grilled chicken and hour-long treadmill sessions. If you are truly depressed, you won't make action your punishment because you won't have the energy to do so. Your form of torture will occur in the mind as you berate yourself for doing such weak and horrible things. We think that if we look in the mirror long enough in disgust, it will get us to avoid the bread basket at dinner; but disgust is an uncomfortable emotion, and you know what feels comforting? Warm bread and butter. The reason your punishment tactics don't work is that deep and lasting change happens only through love, not force. You have to love and respect yourself enough to empower change.

Imagine you get caught talking about a friend behind her back. You know she's pissed, but three days later you ask her if she can pick you up from the airport. Can you picture her response? I assume it's something like, "Hmm...hope you packed light, have fun walking." Now imagine I wake up, walk into the bathroom, and look in the mirror. I say to myself, "Ugh, you fat pig; you have no willpower, you did it again last night, you heifer. You are a flabby, pale before-picture." Then within minutes I start complaining that I can't get my act together, that my body betrays me, and that I can't get away with anything. Why do we think we can talk smack about ourselves and then turn around and do something nice and loving for us? Our bodies want love, they want self-care, they want respect, dammit!

Loving your body is not a lie. You don't have to pretend you are the fittest person in the world. Love can look like acceptance for where you are and a deep desire to move toward where you want to be. You have to start by making peace with your body and by not comparing it to what you don't have. This is your body right now; it is perfectly imperfect. The good news is that most of our hang-ups are completely within our power to change (just not my precious cellulite).

If there is something you don't like that you cannot change, such as your nose, the shape of your eyes, or your voice, then stop putting so much focus on it. I find that the people who are most obsessed with their outer appearance use it as a distraction so as to not have to deal with something deeper within themselves that needs to be worked on. Usually there is something missing in their spiritual life, career, or relationship that truly needs the healing, but since that is too scary to approach without the right tools, flabby arms, thick ankles, or a pointy nose becomes the area of focus.

Create a Peace Treaty

We all have a body part that we notice more than other parts. It's the first thing we see when we try on clothes or look at ourselves naked, that one imperfection that drives us crazy. It's easy to let this negative focus drown out all the positive aspects of you just waiting to be noticed and praised. It's time to put away the fighting words and make a peace treaty with your entire body. Do not skip this important work. I want you to write a letter to your body. (Don't roll your eyes at me! Just trust me.) You probably owe it an apology for being unnecessarily nitpicky and straight-up mean. Once you clear the air and make your amends, create a code of ethics for how you will talk to your physical self. Get specific about the body parts that require a neutral story.

When I see my cellulite in the mirror, my story is, "This is the way my skin attaches to the fascia in this area. That's all it is. It seems it is sticking with me for life, so keep doing those squats and focus on feeling good." I've said that statement so many times that now my focus hardly ever goes to my thighs. I've trained my mind that this is always going to be my response. At this point I think my mind figures, "Why even bother torturing her with the cellulite story; she's just going to say the same thing over and over again, and I'm not getting any drama out of it, so I might as well just move on." Well then, go ahead and do it, lady!

You have to be willing to let go of some of your most deeply ingrained stories. Do it so you can get to a place of camaraderie with yourself. Instead of force, try gentle, loving companionship. Work with, not against, your body. Try being your own best friend. What would you say to her in a moment of vulnerability? What encouragement would you offer? You are committed to improving your health. Let your physical body be the reflection of that focus, not the other way around. While you are letting go of things, let go of the story that this type of relationship shouldn't be this hard. It's not supposed to be easy; you are going against the pattern of the survival mind. Instead say to yourself, "I can understand why this isn't easy, but I'm going to practice until I get there."

Is It Guilt or Is It Shame?

I don't know if it's the Jewish part of me, but unlike practically every psychologist who will tell you that guilt is a useless emotion, I believe it is an incredibly useful tool. If I didn't feel guilt, I would have a closet full of stolen clothes and jewelry from Nordstrom. I would skip out on restaurant tabs when the food is bad, I would sneak into movie theaters without a ticket, and I would most certainly eat dessert for breakfast. I look at the emotion of guilt as any other negative emotion; it's a trigger for me to do some mental work. Guilt is your higher intuitive self saying to you, "Hmm, something's a little off here. Your ethics and morals are being sacrificed, and you might want to take a closer look at this behavior."

If guilt is carrying this kind of message, then it can act as a moral compass, showing you where you veered off track. As useful as this intuitive message is, it's only truly serving you for a few minutes. Any longer than that, and your mind is creating a story that can suck you in, chew you up, and spit you out... directly into the pantry where you hid the cookies in the toaster oven because you thought you might forget that they were there.

One day out of the blue, a contact from Lululemon (an athletic clothes retailer) emailed my assistant, asking to set up a brainstorming meeting. They wanted to collaborate with me to make positive body image signage for their dressing rooms. At first my ego grew several sizes, and I was feeling pretty badass. "So this is what it feels like to be picked first for the soccer team." They wanted me, and I wanted free workout clothes! As the meeting drew closer, my mind went from superior to inferior. "Why did they pick me? I'm not pretty enough or fit enough. Am I cool enough for Lulu?"

When meeting day finally arrived, I picked out my hippest outfit and visualized great success. Although the meeting went well, I could tell I just wasn't myself. I was trying too hard to be funny and cool. I had put them on a pedestal and created a story about not being good enough, so I had to overdo the very things I felt insecure about. As soon as they walked out the door, I felt this pang in my stomach. I knew what it was; I knew the feeling well, it was guilt. My intuitive voice was saying, "Carly, you fugged up, girlfriend. You didn't need to be anything more than who you are." I ignored the message and distracted myself with other work.

Over the next few days, I would have flashbacks to a joke I made that returned no laughter or a story I told that was slightly enhanced, and I would physically cringe. I would cringe in the shower while I was shampooing my hair, I would cringe in the car at the stoplight, and I would cringe while peeing, which is when I do all my good thinking. Think about a time you did something you weren't proud of (or "did" someone you weren't proud of) and how long that feeling of regret and guilt followed you. This is the perfect example of when guilt is *not* useful. Of when the mind takes over and sucks you in. If I had given myself space to do a little reflection when I first felt the pang in my stomach, I would have rewritten the story, learned my lesson, and moved on with clarity. Instead, I let guilt fester into shame by allowing my monkey mind to take the reins.

According to well-known shame researcher Brené Brown, *guilt* is defined as the feeling that you have engaged in wrong or bad behavior. Shame, on the other hand, is the story you tell yourself that who you *are* is wrong. If you finish the chapter on conscious eating and then eat too much at dinner, you might feel a little guilty because your behavior was not in alignment with how you wanted to honor your body's communication around food. If you overeat at dinner and then call yourself a stupid pig, now you are allowing the behavior to create your identity, who you believe you are. This is shame. Who you believe you are at your core gets confused with something you did, and this is a slippery slope, one that you do not want to go down.

I would never want you or anyone else to judge yourself on your worst day or at your worst moment. Similarly, I don't want you to judge your worst body part. It's not who you are; it's how you look. It's not who you are; it's how you ate during that one meal. It's not who you are; it's how you acted when you were feeling insecure. Although I acted fake and insecure in the meeting, that's not who I am when I am holding myself in the highest regard. It was simply a behavior based on my unhelpful story of not feeling like I was enough. Separating your true sense of self from your behaviors (and most-hated body parts) makes forgiveness and growth a whole lot easier. I wound up getting the Lululemon gig despite my corny jokes and exaggerated stories. Or maybe those jokes got me the gig. Either way, Lulu helped me far more than I helped them, because this experience helped me grow a little more beyond my ego's silly stories.

End the Battle and Become an Expert Negotiator

When my nephew was three and a half, I made the dire mistake of bringing him with me to Target. I was trying to help my sister out by babysitting and help myself out by checking errands off the list at the same time. In what was truly a rookie maneuver, I pushed the cart past the toy aisle without giving it a second thought. Wouldn't you know that the exact millisecond that his eye caught the first glimpse of primary-colored plastic he morphed into Stretch Armstrong, reached out his rubbery arm, and grabbed onto the first toy his sticky little fingers could touch. Of course, I was under explicit instructions from my sister not to buy him anything, so there we stood, two soldiers at the front line, ready to battle it out over some five-dollar piece of plastic junk.

Naturally, my nephew used his best weapon and starting throwing a temper tantrum. I immediately scanned the area to see what parents would meet my eyes and give me the reassuring "this is not your fault" nod, but sadly I was met with judgmental "control your child" side-eye only. I wanted to scream, "He's not mine! I'm just the aunt! Fine, he's a spoiled little brat!" but then I quickly decided that it wouldn't help me and moved into self-preservation mode. That led me to wonder whether I could just rip the toy out of his hand and run out of the store, but if you have ever tried to put a wailing toddler in a car seat, you know that this was not a viable option. I couldn't battle this one out. The only option I had was to get down on his level, understand his viewpoint, and negotiate.

You know what toddlers love? Instant gratification. Their world revolves around it. They don't care that a doughnut will ruin their dinner or give them a bellyache; they want sweet satisfaction right now. Sound familiar? Your inner fat kid is eternally three years old. You can try to yell at yourself, force yourself, hate yourself enough to create change, but your body and mind will react like a toddler clutching a toy in Target. You might win a battle or two, but ultimately you lose the long fight. Instead, you have to get down to your own level, create some self-compassion, and negotiate new terms. I told my nephew that I understood he wanted the toy. I added that if he would quiet down, we could go home and read books together and cuddle, his favorite activity, next to eating doughnuts.

If you are craving junk, don't immediately shame yourself for the craving. Agree with yourself; why wouldn't you want to eat something so delicious and easy? Why, yes, eating popcorn mindlessly on the couch could help you zone out and give you a break from reality. Why don't you make tea tonight and take a hot shower, then on Friday night, lovingly make yourself a popcorn treat, rent a movie, and enjoy it with intention? Stop basing your food choices on who wins the angel-and-devil saga: "I want it; no, I shouldn't have it; but screw it, who cares; no, you will regret this..." and start having a real conversation with yourself, a conversation that fosters a loving relationship between you, your body, and your mind.

Healthy Striving vs. Perfectionism

Our most destructive eating behaviors stem from this kind of black-and-white mentality. Either you will eat perfectly, or you will wait until tomorrow to try again, which means you have until the end of the day to go absolutely crazy because, hey, you already failed, so you might as well have fun! The same thing goes for our bodies. For those of us who have a lot of weight to lose, we think we are so far from the finish line that what's the point of even trying? If you fall into the category of wanting to lose the last five to ten nagging pounds, you might find yourself nitpicking the tiniest imperfections. Even though the weight-loss goal of a hundred pounds feels worlds away from five pounds, people in both categories may find themselves stuck in the prison of striving to achieve perfection.

Healthy striving conjures up the question, "How can I improve?" It allows you to push yourself a little bit each day while resetting in the moment when needed. It's a question that brings us inside, asking our internal guide how to make the next step in growth. Perfectionism, on the other hand, asks, "What will others think?" If you want your body, or your personality, to be perfect, it's because you are viewing yourself through the eyes of others. No matter who validates you, there will always be someone who will tear you down, and that will be the one person your mind decides to listen to. You are not everyone's cup of tea or perfect 10. The other day I met someone who despises Ellen DeGeneres. My first thought was "You must be insane. Who hates Ellen? Anyone who hates Ellen probably also hates cats and finds Oprah, with all her do-gooder-ness, annoying."

Accept that no matter how healthy and fit you are, the human body will always have its imperfections. Remember, the perfect bodies you see on social media and in magazines have been airbrushed, and as for the 1 percent of women who were genetically blessed to have the body our culture deems perfect, well, I'm sure they have horrible breath and recurring yeast infections. All kidding aside, even these women have something they don't like about themselves. It may not be physical, but they might think they aren't smart enough or worry that they aren't doing something meaningful enough with their lives. There will always be something, which is great because it gives us opportunities to practice acceptance.

Skimmer's Delight

✓ Body image and dieting are directly related. You can't heal one without healing the other.
✓ Your standard of physical beauty needs to come from a place of self-love, not out of an attempt at worthiness.
✓ Guilt is a very useful emotion — but if it lasts for longer than a minute, your egoic mind has taken over.
✓ You are your own best friend and number one cheerleader.
✓ Healthy striving creates the path to enlightenment. Perfection is concerned only with what others think.

Make It Stick

1. Create five letting-go statements:

   When I'm willing to let go of __________, then I will finally be able to accomplish or feel __________.

2. Write yourself a letter and create a peace treaty. Make amends and move forward with a new set of standards for how you will treat and talk to yourself.
3. Create a list of ten things you love about your body and your inner self. Say these to yourself every time you look in the mirror.

chapter 9

LIFE IS BEST WHEN YOU MANIFEST

Believe that you have it, and you have it.
— Latin proverb

Imagination is a much stronger force than willpower.
— Claude Bristol

How much time do you spend focusing on the body you have versus the body you want? When you look in the mirror, is it hard to imagine that you would ever feel pride, love, and respect for what's reflected back at you? This hopeless feeling can reach far beyond your body. It's easily applied to your bank account, your relationship, your living situation, your wardrobe, and so on. Sometimes we feel so far from our goal that we don't believe we will ever achieve success. It's that very story that can lead us down the path of destruction: "I'm so far from where I want to be, what's this one bite / sip / entire pizza to myself going to do?"

It's easy to get stuck when you are focused on how far you have to go to reach the finish line. I hate to get all Debbie Downer on you, but deep down, we both know that there is no such thing as a finish line when it comes to your health. Once you get into peak health and physical fitness, it takes daily effort to stay there. The good news is that you are already doing all the things needed to keep it up! If you are feeling daily discouragement, odds are you are missing this key component to creating the life and body you want: the art of manifesting.

Martin Luther King Jr., Mahatma Gandhi, Marie Curie, Thomas Edison, Maya Angelou, the Wright Brothers, Amelia Earhart: They all believed in their vision with such intensity and certainty that they willed it into existence. They proved that it is our innate human power to think beyond our current reality. They lived their vision as if it was going to happen. Through conviction, they proved the magic of belief.

This chapter will teach you how to stop seeing your body, and current state of health, as a hopeless disappointment and begin to see it as how you want it to be. The ability to manifest your vision for ultimate health and happiness is one of the most overlooked tools in creating permanent change. Most of us stopped using our imaginations a long time ago and have become ignorant to the power that lies within us, the power to shape our reality.

Finally, Proof That Turns Woo-Woo into Science

Mystics, sages, healers, and patchouli-smelling hippies have been teaching this magic for thousands of years. The only problem was that they couldn't prove it scientifically. Manifestation, the concept that you have the power to write your own story with the vibration put out by your thoughts and emotions, was a lovely theory backed by many anecdotal stories, but, the skeptics asked, where was the proof?

In the early 1900s, the skeptics received their answer through the discovery of quantum physics. Joe Dispenza, an expert in neurology, neuroscience, and cellular biology, explained the fundamental concept of quantum physics by stating, "All potential experiences exist in the quantum field as a sea of infinite possibilities. When you change your electromagnetic signature [by changing how you think and feel] to match one that already exists in the field, your body will be drawn to that event, you will move into a new line of time, or the event will find you in your new reality." His studies proved that thinking in new ways, as well as changing beliefs, can help you not only to rewire the human brain but also to make your dreams and desires a reality.

Before you feel the need to smoke a joint to help you understand this concept, I will break it down for you while you are still sober (or if you've already smoked, strap in and get ready to expand your mind, man). Science can now measure, through wavelengths, the energy that we emit with our thoughts and emotions. These wavelengths, also called vibrations, draw similar experiences into your life. We are energetically calling in our present-day reality by what we are thinking and feeling. We are creating our destiny and fulfilling our prophecies. Instead of changing our external environment, quantum physics proves that we can change our internal environment (thoughts and emotions) to create change in our outside world.

Our thoughts not only manifest our reality, but they also are responsible for our quality of life. Every time you have a thought, the mind sends the body a chemical message (through neurotransmitters) that says "because you are thinking this thought, you should feel this way." In turn, the body releases hormones that send a signal back to the brain to let the brain know the body is now feeling exactly how the brain is thinking. This feedback loop is almost simultaneous and a beautiful example of how positive thinking can make us feel happy and at peace. It can also be a vicious circle when negative thinking creates an emotional stress response, which confirms to the mind that its fear-based thoughts were correct and that we do in fact have something to feel bad about.

Mental Rehearsal

So often we focus on the things we don't want without realizing that we are calling forth those exact experiences into our lives. The minute you buy airline tickets, you hope the flight won't get delayed. Once you decide on a restaurant, you wonder whether or not there will be a long wait. A week after you start a new diet or workout, you wonder how long it will be before you fall off the wagon. We know that the mind is set up this way to ensure its most basic survival; however, in our modern world, where a water buffalo is never coming to stomp down our mud hut, it is doing us more harm than good.

One of the key steps in manifesting the health and body you desire is to mentally rehearse living in that body. Mental rehearsal is a crucial tool for letting go of old patterns and moving toward what you deserve. Instead of thinking about your body the way it is, I want you to practice thinking (and feeling) about it the way you want it to be.

Try setting a timer for three minutes in the morning. During those three minutes, I want you to visualize living in the body you want. What would it feel like to wake up in the best shape and the best health of your life? How do you move through the day? What are you wearing, what are you thinking, how do you interact with people? What do you eat, how do you hold yourself, what are you experiencing? Remember, you have to feel this in the body. When I'm manifesting, I know that I'm feeling it when the corners of my mouth start to curl. My face physically reacts to the emotions coursing through my body.

Thoughts and Feelings Have to Match

Have you ever tried to manifest something in your life, all the while feeling like it wasn't going to happen? We put out mixed signals all the time. We repeat positive affirmations about financial abundance; then we feel anxious when we open our bills or look at our bank accounts. We visualize meeting the perfect partner but sit on the couch depressed, wondering if our destiny is to be the crazy cat woman who talks to herself at the bus stop. We desire to live in a radiant body that we are proud of, but we nitpick every imperfection the second we see ourselves in the mirror. You might think abundant thoughts but feel scarcity around every facet of your life: money, time, food, your body, and your relationships.

Words are a great start, but if you intend to put out a strong electromagnetic signal that pulls you toward the future you want, you must think of your thoughts as simply a support to your emotions. If your emotions are the signal, your thoughts are the catalyst to get those good-vibe juices flowin'.

Gratitude Is the Best Attitude

If the name of the manifestation game is to feel as if your dream has already become a reality, then a great tool for getting you to feel the accomplishment of your vision is to live in a state of gratitude as much as humanly possible. When you wake up, thank the Universe for already having an amazing, productive day. When you think about what you want, say "thank you" as if you have already received it. When you think about your ideal body, give thanks for the strength that it takes to make all the best choices at the moment they arise.

A practice that instantly puts me in a feel-good mood, and allows me to put out the vibration to receive all that I'm manifesting, is to wish for others to be happy. When I call the customer service of any company, right as he asks if he can assist with anything else, I say a silent prayer wishing him to be happy. When I swipe my credit card at a pharmacy, grocery store, or any other random place, I look at the cashier and picture her laughing, surrounded by friends or family, and I silently wish for her to have peace and happiness. Try this yourself. This practice will put you in a great-feeling place, since you are giving out the same electromagnetic abundance that you are calling to manifest into your own life. Try it for a week; walk around dropping love bombs all over the place and see what it does to your emotional disposition.

Don't Complain

This is a tough one because, oh man, do we love to complain, about traffic, the weather, our aching pinkie toes, our annoying mothers-in-law, roommates, and whatever else we can possibly harp on! This morning I found myself complaining that the big forks in my cutlery are too big and heavy. I mean, seriously? What, did my hand stop working? I suggest you try going one full day without complaining about anything. You might think that's an easy task, and you would be a stronger person than I am. In fact, I've been sitting in this same exact chair for three hours now, and my butt kinda hurts. Whoops, there I go again.

You will be relieved to know that there is a certain amount of lag time when it comes to manifestation, which means that anytime you catch yourself in a negative cycle of thinking, you still have time to correct it. I was taught that one positive thought can negate two negative ones. It may sound corny, but if you think about it, it makes sense. Consider the idea that one sincere thought of gratitude can neutralize two self-centered complaints. This belief allows us to be human, to make a mistake, and to still have the ability to correct it. In the same way that we can relive the past by playing it over and over again in our minds, we can also manifest the future.

I don't want you to miss a beat when it comes to taking ownership of your quality of life. Creating the changes you want, and making them stick, is going to require much more than eating vegetables and exercising. Using the mind to work on your behalf puts you on the road to guaranteeing that the life you want is the life you are living!

Skimmer's Delight

- ✓ The Universe is a place of "yes." Whatever you want to manifest, it says yes to. What are you putting out there?

- ✓ The most important key to manifesting all that you desire is to think and feel the way you would if you already had received the abundance you are calling in.
- ✓ The rules for manifesting the body you want are mentally rehearse; ensure that your thoughts and feelings match; have gratitude as if what you desire has already come to you; and don't complain.
- ✓ To manifest at your highest capacity, you have to be vibrating at a high frequency. Gratitude and love will get you there every time.
- ✓ Fear and gratitude cannot live in your heart and mind at the same time.

Make It Stick

Write down a list of three things you would like to manifest. Take a few moments to visualize what it would look and feel like for you to have these things, people, and experiences in your life. Take three minutes every morning to do your manifestation exercise!

chapter 10

THE TRAINED MIND

enroll in mental boot camp

The mind is the source of all suffering,
and it is also the source of all happiness. — **Pema Chödrön**

We are shaped by our thoughts; we become what we think.
When the mind is pure, joy follows like a shadow that never leaves.
— **Buddha**

You have power over your mind, not outside events.
Realize this, and you will find strength. — **Marcus Aurelius**

What if I told you that you could train yourself to become not only physically strong but emotionally strong as well? Just as you train your muscles to withstand stress, you can train your mind to withstand the emotional stress that would otherwise throw you off your health and happiness game. This means that you are in charge of your emotions, not other people, not situations, not past hurts, not objects. Since all negative behaviors stem from emotions that we don't manage, becoming emotionally strong means that you have complete control over what winds up on your plate. Food loses its illusory power, and you find a level of inner strength and wisdom that you never knew you had.

Like any strength training, this will be difficult. What's even harder is that just when you think you have the hang of it, the Universe will throw a curveball your way and knock you on your ass. I've been intentionally training my mind for years, and some moments I feel as emotionally strong as an animal lover watching one of those ten-minute-long ASPCA commercials. Emotions do pass, thank goodness, and those weak moments give me an opportunity to take inventory on the places where I can improve. By doing that work, I grow, and that is always a good thing. I'm going to share with you my best tools for returning to a state of emotional strength and power. Just promise me that you will be gentle with yourself. As you begin this practice, know that your humanness guarantees a sliding scale of success. Some days will be better than others. If you commit to this practice, trust that over time you will find more ease in taking back your emotions and living in an empowered, grateful, and peaceful state.

Best-Case-Scenario Thinking

When we discussed the three ways we get into stress in chapter 4 (which is worth a double read if you are prone to anxiety), you learned that one of the ways we lose control of our emotions is when the mind conjures up the worst-possible future scenario and then tortures us with that possibility even though it's (1) not what we want and (2) not even happening. If you are enrolling in mental boot camp, you must decide, from here on out, to identify as a best-case-scenario thinker.

This means that in any situation, you remind yourself to visualize the best-possible scenario. I don't want you to focus on a "pretty good outcome." I want you to shoot for the stars! Be greedy and conjure up the ideal story line for your movie. Spielberg it up, because let's face it, we all deserve to kiss DiCaprio at the end! Anytime I find myself feeling emotionally low, I know that I am not focusing on what I want. As my meditation teacher told me, worrying is like praying for something you don't want. Now that you are well studied in the art of manifestation, you realize that best-case-scenario thinking is not only the way to create your ideal reality but also a mental mainline to feeling emotionally strong in the present moment, even before the future has presented itself.

All you need is this one question: "What would be the absolute best-case scenario here?" This tells the mind to go right where you want it, focusing on the positive. What you focus on, you feel. This one question contains the ultimate power. It simply trains the mind to focus on your real solution instead of on the problem at hand.

Trigger Emotions

If you want to train the mind, you need to change the way you experience negative emotions. Instead of getting stuck in them, you begin to see those bad feelings as trigger emotions. They are triggering you to do the spiritual work needed to grow as an individual who is seeking a life of ease and abundance. It's not that we shouldn't experience negative emotions; it's that we shouldn't dwell on them. Trigger emotions are there for a good reason, but they are only useful for a moment (much like guilt). Once you feel bad, that's your cue to think, "Okay, something is up. Time to do some inquiry." Inquiry entails a set of questions that you ask yourself to get to the bottom of what thoughts are causing you to feel bad. Here are some questions to ask yourself when you become aware that you are in a disempowered emotional state.

When you are upset by the actions of others:

- What is this really about?
- What is my story here, and what part is causing me suffering?
- Is there any illusion here that I can rewrite?

- If this were not about anyone else but me, what would this situation reflect about me that I need to work on?

When you are feeling anxious or depressed:

- What positive core belief would help me see this differently?
- Am I succumbing to one of the three pitfalls of stress/fear?
- What's my ideal outcome? How can I control this outcome?
- What do I need to let go of?
- Which emotion do I need to bring forth in this moment? Is it the spiritual practice of patience, love, respect, surrender, compassion, and/or awareness?

Although I categorized these questions, any one of them can help you in any situation in which you find yourself being controlled by the mind. After you do the mental work and come up with your solution, I'd like you to go back to the five core beliefs I shared with you on page 30 (or the ones you made up on your own) and solidify your mental training with the best-matched core belief to prove your new story to be true. Notice that with this work, you used a negative trigger emotion to get you back to a place of experiencing mental clarity and peacefulness. Are you able to see these negative emotions as a guide to help you get back into the positive?

How many times a day will you have to do this work? Maybe a hundred, if you are lucky. If you commute, your practice will probably start when you're in morning traffic. You will subconsciously be thinking about how late you will be and who will judge you when you walk into the office (focusing on things you can't control, making things worse than they are, dress-rehearsing the worst-case scenario: congrats, mind; you have successfully employed all three ways we lose control of our emotions by letting fear/stress take power, and this was all before your morning coffee kicked in! Isn't the mind impressive?).

In this situation, what question from above works the best for your commuter soul search?

Truthfully, you could use all of them, but if it were me, and we both know that this is a "me" kinda move, I would ask myself, "What is this really about?" The immediate answer would be, "I'm worrying that other people would feel like I am not enough. I'm not punctual enough, I don't care about my job enough, I'm not motivated enough," and so on. Once I recognize that the "not-enough" story is dragging me down, I go to my core beliefs and pull out two of my big guns: "Everything is unfolding perfectly because, you know what? I'll get there when I get there! I am enough, and the Universe has my back." The best-case scenario is that traffic lightens up, and I walk in right on time. Better yet, no one is around when I get there because they are all stuck in traffic too! Now look who's early!

Fast-forward to the end of the day. (I assume you have now done this mental training a hundred times between the time you were stuck in traffic and the present, when you are finally home and able to relax on the couch.) You are exhausted, and you are craving something sweet as a reward for working your butt off all day. That craving of yours is a trigger emotion; notice that it doesn't feel good to crave something unhealthy when you want to improve your health. You start to feel a little anxious because you don't feel strong enough to simply witness the craving without action. You can feel that you are about to cave. Time to do the work. Which question from the above list would best guide you back to a place of power over the mind? Again, any of these great inquiry probes would work, but for this example, I'm going to use these: "What's my ideal outcome? What is it I truly want? How can I control this outcome? What do I need to let go of?"

My ideal outcome is to wake up tomorrow feeling proud of myself that I made the best decisions for my health and didn't use food as comfort. What I want is to eat when I'm hungry and find ways to self-soothe that are all reward and no consequence. I can control this outcome by deciding to floss and brush or just make some soothing hot tea. I need to let go of the illusion that eating at night comforts me. In truth, it creates a body that I am not comfortable in.

It may sound exhausting to do all this mind work all the time, but I want you to realize that your mind is at work all the time anyway. You are simply taking back power and training the mind to think the way you want it to so that you can feel good and then act in accordance with those higher-level emotions. You are essentially taking the same energy you would if you just let the mind go wild. Think about how exhausting it is to go back and forth on whether or not to eat the cookie. The mind is running; you are simply using tools to steer it in the right direction.

Process vs. Outcome

Do you need to lose a substantial amount of weight or just a few pounds? Are you trying to heal the pain in your body? Do you want to make a major change in any aspect of your life, whether it be your relationships, your job, or your living situation? Regardless of your particular desire, the single most powerful mental thing you can do is to train your mind to immediately focus on the desired outcome rather than on the process.

It's Jennifer's first appointment at Nutritional Wisdom, and we are going over her vision of optimal health. Her goals are to lose weight and feel super confident in a bikini, have energy that lasts all day, get through the cold season without getting sick, and gain the confidence to leave her current job and go for the career of her dreams.

As we talk more and I ask her to explain what her life would be like as a result of achieving these things, her face lights up, and she becomes really animated. "I would have the most amazing life! I would truly feel like I was able to give the world all I have to offer and get the most out of life in return!" I continue to push her. "How else would achieving these goals improve your quality of life?" "I would put myself out there more, and I imagine I would finally meet my life partner, travel the world, and have a family. Then I could experience true love and adventure!" At this point, Jennifer is so focused on her outcome that she is willing to do anything necessary to make it happen.

Now imagine if once Jennifer shared her goals with me, I immediately jumped into the process of what she will need to do to achieve them. "Well, Jennifer, these are fantastic goals. Let's talk about how to get you there. First of all, you need to cut sugar, dairy, gluten, and alcohol from your diet 80 percent of the time. This means you probably need new friends, or better yet, just don't have any friends at all. You need to spend a few hours a week in the kitchen cooking your foods. Oh, yes, and you will have to food shop once a week and wash a ton of dishes. You will need to work out four to five times a week, which means you will be doing a lot of laundry in your free time. You also need to drink more water than you ever imagined possible and remember to swallow those horse pill–size supplements every day. You will need to budget for this, because health takes time and money, two things you probably don't feel like you have enough of. By the way, however early you've been waking up, you probably need to get up an hour earlier so you can chop onions and garlic, and empty the dishwasher from the night before."

I could go on, but I'd be talking to myself because Jennifer has already grabbed her purse and run right out the door! She's heading straight to the closest fast-food joint to stuff her face with fries because the process is way too painful and overwhelming — that is, without remembering what is truly at stake. Whatever your vision for optimal health is, make sure that every day you train the mind to focus on the desired outcome. The one question I ask myself more than anything else is, "What is my ideal outcome?"

Watch Your Language

It was a particularly unpleasant day outside: gray, muggy, and pouring. Somehow I willed myself to go to a yoga class. In most yoga classes, before we start moving, the teacher usually gives a little intro to help the class set an intention. At the beginning of her intro on that morning she said, "I love days like this. What an awesome, nourishing day for all the plants!" I thought to myself, "This lady has lost her mind. It's nasty out, and this weather makes me want to crawl under a blanket and do nothing." After I let it sink in a bit, I thought, "Well, she does look a lot happier and more content than I am right now. I guess she's right. It's been super hot and dry here, and today is a nice break from the heat, not only for the plants but for me too." It was a small moment of clarity, but I realized that I hadn't chosen to think negatively about the weather; my untrained mind had just gone to the negative without my catching it. I could have woken up loving whatever weather was happening if I was just conscious enough to choose my words carefully.

Focus and language are of utmost importance when you have enrolled your mind in mental optimism boot camp. We know that what you focus on you feel and that your language dictates your focus. You see, there's always going to be something wrong in your day, in your world, with the world, in your relationships, and so on. There's also always going to be something right. It is your language that sets the tone.

Just the other day I caught myself thinking about how overwhelmed I was. My mind kept reminding me how much I had to do. It just loves to turn a gift into a problem. The things I need to do are a gift in my life. They create the abundance that I experience each day. My mind, however, was trying its hardest to turn that blessing into a problem. Its uninvited commentary tried to convince me that there was just too much that needed to be done. I simply changed my language and put an end to the overwhelming story. I kept repeating over and over again, "It always gets done, I always get it done, all at the right time, this is a gift." Never forget that words carry tremendous power. They can put you in a place of darkness or in a state of peace. You have complete control over one of the most powerful forces in your life. Now, that's a true gift!

Ask the Right Questions

While I have your mind laser-focused on language, let's discuss the power of asking high-quality questions. The mind is constantly conjuring up questions as you move through the day. The sad truth is that the mind prefers to think up problem-focused questions. Problem-focused questions lead you toward an answer that has no room for a solution. These questions aren't questions at all; they are judgments made with a raised voice and a question mark at the end. They keep you stuck in what's wrong and are pretty useless, if you ask me. "Did I just say that?! What is wrong with me?"

Your higher self offers solution-based questions, which leave room for new insight and creativity. They allow room for multiple answers to be explored, and they take you to a new level of understanding and therefore massive right action! Here are a few of the most common problem- vs. solution-based questions. As you read through them, notice how different your answer is based on where the wording of the question prompts you to put your focus.

Problem-Based vs. Solution-Based Questions

Problem-Based	*Solution-Based*
Why do I have this problem?	What can I learn from this?
What is wrong with me?	What is my main focus for improvement?
How can I get more?	How can I find even more enjoyment with what I already have?
What is wrong with people?	How can I be more compassionate in this instance?
Why can't I get my shit together?	What is the first step I can take to heal this pattern?
Why is it so hard?	What limiting belief, if reframed, could help make this easy?

Next time you catch the mind asking a question, make sure the answer is one that helps you move forward. If you don't like your answer, then think about your ideal solution and ask yourself a higher-quality question.

When All Else Fails

Regardless of the external circumstance, these tools usually allow me to get my mind and body back to a place of peace, heightened inner awareness, and gratitude. However, sometimes I use every tool in my pink, bedazzled toolbox, and the negative feelings still stick. Maybe the incident is just too fresh, my stories too strong. Sometimes I can admit that while on the surface I am trying to change my perspective, deep down inside I'm not yet ready, and for the love of all things drama, my mind is wanting me to stay stuck a little longer. Regardless of the reason, it's guaranteed that I will find myself feeling shitty and wanting to sleep, eat, and shop my problems away. If you find yourself in this place, and your tools aren't working (or you aren't feeling able to use them), the best thing to do is to interrupt your mental pattern by changing your physiology.

I could be in the worst mood, and you could change it in an instant by blasting some '90s pop music. I wouldn't be able to help myself; my body would tell my bad attitude to take a hike as I rocked out to TLC telling me not to chase any more waterfalls. The music wouldn't solve any of my problems; only I have the power to do that. What it would do is interrupt my thought pattern and change my physiology. Author Tony Robbins always says that "motion moves emotion." If you can't work your stories, you can move your body to move stuck emotions so that they can easily pass right through you. Music may not always be appropriate for the situation, especially when dealing with shock or trauma. Talking a walk in nature helps me when I'm in the most distress. While I walk, I take long, deep breaths and try to stay really present to whatever is around me. Even crying is a vehicle for driving out stinky, sticky emotions. So often after I cry, even though I haven't begun to do the work, I feel a little relieved.

Interrupting your emotional pattern with a physical change in your body allows you to press the reset button. Exercising, walking, dancing, or punching a pillow with all-out effort: all these things will help you get unstuck. Afterward, check back in with yourself and see if you are willing and able to do some mind work on the subject at hand. If you are still stuck, just say a simple prayer to your higher self: "Please help me be willing to let this go, to do the work needed, and to free myself so I can be at peace." With time, you will be able to use these tools to get back in control of the voice in your head. Peaceful energy then extends itself to your dinner plate and beyond.

Skimmer's Delight

- ✓ Just as you train your muscles to withstand stress, you can train your mind to withstand the emotional stress that would otherwise throw you off your health and happiness game.
- ✓ Best-case-scenario thinking is not only the way to create your ideal reality but also an immediate pathway toward feeling emotionally strong in the present moment.
- ✓ Trigger emotions are there to help guide you back to a place of feeling good. Use them to recognize that you need to do some mental work.
- ✓ Regardless of the particular desire, the single most powerful mental tool you can employ is to train your mind to immediately focus on your desired outcome rather than on the process.
- ✓ We know that what you focus on you feel, and your language dictates your focus.

✓ When all else fails, interrupt your mental pattern by changing your physiology.

Make It Stick

1. List the top three trigger emotions you feel daily. For each emotion, list a set of questions you can ask to guide yourself back to feeling emotionally strong. Write about how you will look at these emotions as a gift to help you do the long-term work of controlling the mind.
2. Give an example of something you would often think or say that disempowers you. Use empowering language to shift your focus to what you want. Take these words and make them your daily mantra.
3. Describe a situation in which you tend to focus on the process instead of on the desired outcome. Write a brief but strongly worded phrase to help guide yourself, with focused, positive mental language, toward the desired outcome.

chapter 11

FINALLY FULFILLED

Soon your frustration will outgrow your resistance,
and at that point, change will happen. — **Me**

Anyone who has had weight-loss success has also had failure.
Think of it as your badge of honor, and don't judge what phase you are in.
— **Me again**

It is so incredibly easy to get sucked into the illusion that weight loss is all about food. The logical mind thinks, "Why wouldn't it be? What I eat is causing my weight gain, so this must be about food." This story initiates the quest to try every diet out there, in order to get your body to a place where you feel "good enough." Confident. Worthy. Desired. Happy. We believe the lie that as long as we fit the physical mold of what our culture deems attractive we will be content. In the world of internal belief systems, this is a dangerous combo, and it doesn't even need to be supersized to pose a threat. The story on loop is the following: if we fit the perfect physical mold, we will live a life of happiness. If we need to lose a few pounds to fit ourselves in, figuratively and literally (wait, who shrunk this thing over the winter?), then we have no choice but to put all our attention and focus on food.

What happens when the diet doesn't work? We make it about us. We failed, we have no willpower, we don't deserve it, we will never get there. We make it about our bodies. They just aren't the same as they used to be, they are stubborn, they are broken and don't work correctly. If you were asked to build a house and had inadequate training for doing so (lack of wisdom of your body's unique nutritional needs) and bad building materials (a mind that controls you), would it be your fault if the roof started leaking (a body that doesn't reflect self-love and deep inner fulfillment)?

The tools in this book all lead you toward a life in which you feel truly fulfilled. To be fulfilled means that you are utterly and deeply filled with the love and adventure life has to offer you. You control the voice in your head so that your higher self calls the shots in your life, *you* rule how you want to live from a place of deep inner wisdom, and you do so with gratitude, courage, and the perfect recipe of piss and vinegar. You realize that each day is a gift, and you become deeply filled by all the little beautiful moments, hidden blessings, and tiny daily miracles. You start to fill up spiritually, so you no longer need to mindlessly fill yourself up physically, with food. Food becomes a part of the way you experience life, but it is in balance, as are the other pleasures in your life.

When you no longer believe the chattering of the monkey mind, you know that the message it's constantly trying to convey to you that you are not enough is not true. You don't need to fill that feeling of not-enoughness with a bowl of popcorn or three hours of nightly TV. You start to crave living life to the fullest. You stop craving food, which, when abused, will dull you and prevent you from living each day in a peaceful, energetic state. When you practice your new core beliefs, life gets easier, and so does healthy eating. Happy people are healthy people.

But what *about* food? Does being spiritually fulfilled automatically make you repulsed by greasy, fried, sugary fare? Of course not. Let's not get crazy here. Those foods are still delicious and delight the senses, in the right environment. What fulfillment *does* do is take the power away from food. It neutralizes our obsession with it. It doesn't make a particular food bad or good. It's just food. Some foods will make us feel better than others, but when food loses its power, we can make logical decisions about how often we want to put certain foods into our bodies, and we can make those decisions based on the knowledge of how these foods will make us feel afterward.

Back when I was at war with my body and therefore was totally obsessed with food, vacations always used to magnify the grossness of my inner vulnerability and chaos. I would go on a crash diet before the vacation to get as lean as possible — no carbs or sugar for this bikini body! Then I would plan the entire vacation around the junk I was going to eat. A classic case of the pendulum swing from food prison to reckless abandonment. About halfway through the vacation, I would feel bloated and tired and would drag throughout the day, energy zapped by all the crappy food my body wasn't used to digesting.

Once I started to take control of my mind, my stress levels lowered. Less stress meant more space to take care of myself, and in doing that I started to notice more beauty in each day. I started smiling more, I was playful, and my emotional state allowed me to attract better experiences into my life. For the first time I started to look at my relationship with food for what it was: simply a mirror for where I was on my spiritual path. The more I controlled my stories and leaned on my new beliefs, the healthier my relationship with food became.

After a few years of doing this work, I found myself on the foodie vacation of a lifetime, a honeymoon to Italy. The land of gluten, dairy, and sugar, my old Achilles' heels, Italy was a perfectly set stage for me to go hog wild. I made it okay to eat whatever I wanted, but I set very strong intentions for honoring my hunger cues and not eating when I wasn't hungry. I was going to consciously eat my way through Italy, and whatever I weighed when I came home was going to be okay with me!

During this trip the most miraculous, beautiful, unexpected thing happened. After the first two days of eating gluten and dairy at every meal, I woke up on day three not wanting that kind of food. I had removed the mental shackles and made myself feel totally free to eat whatever I wanted. With that newfound food freedom, I ultimately just wanted to feel good. After the first few meals, I could feel my energy lowering, I hadn't pooped, and I woke up both mornings with a stomachache. The meals were delicious and certainly worth it, but I had had enough. Throughout the rest of the trip, I ate the most delicious fresh fish and vegetables, with a smattering of bread and gelato here and there. I came home from the trip and weighed myself, and I hadn't gained a pound. It wasn't because I was eating clean; I had something not on my regular food protocol every single day. It was a combo of conscious eating and all-day-long movement that kept me steady at the same weight. The weight wasn't the victory, even though that used to be the only thing that mattered to me. The weight was a reflection of the more important inner victory: I had made these food decisions out of love, not out of fear or by force; I still enjoyed myself as a total foodie; I did not feel restricted; I experienced so much more than the food on the trip, that I was completely present to be fulfilled by it all.

The lack of postvacation weight gain was a plus, even though I would have felt just as victorious returning home a few pounds heavier. I want you to go on vacation, enjoy yourself, eat foods you normally wouldn't eat, drink more than you normally would, and enjoy life while maintaining the balance of still feeling good. Don't let food keep you from enjoying something greater being offered to you. Come home from vacation and get right back into the groove. If your body goes up and down five pounds, don't give it another thought. Soak in as much of life as you can, which includes the famous fried cheese-stuffed squash blossom in Italy or the sought-after funnel cake on the pier at your childhood summer vacation spot (which will mean so much more to you than that pint of ice cream on your couch any night of the week).

There is a natural zigzag-shaped path to health that creates ultimate balance without forcing you to sacrifice your health or physical image. You zig a little so you can experience eating foods without boundary, foods that light up your senses in a way that other foods can't in that moment. Then you rebound back to what will eventually feel normal, healthy, and minimally effortful. Healthy living will always require effort, but over time that effort feels natural; it is the foundation on which you build your best life. Unhealthy eating feels more like a binge diet than your protein and veggies do, and when you experience that, you have made a true food transformation.

On vacation, it may look like eating dinner out every night but also like taking a taxi to a trusted grocery store as soon as you get there, so that you can stock up on some salads and healthy snacks for in between. During a normal week, it may look like going out to eat and drink with friends on one or two nights, but let's not forget that you've been batch-cooking and exercising most of the week. No food should be off-limits to you (unless avoiding it is required for healing). You always have to give yourself that choice and the opportunity to reset if, when looking back on the day, you see that you didn't make the best decision.

Despite all our hard work, we are still human, and we are still imperfect. We will make mistakes, old patterns will pop up when we least expect them, and the occasional binge will remind us that this life is a practice, not a perfect. For this reason, we need to learn how to forgive instantly, authentically, and with a tremendous amount of compassion. We are going to do, say, and eat things that make us cringe. Stories will come back about how unworthy we are, and we need to be ready to forgive, learn, and move forward with a new sense of clarity.

When I ask people to be gentler on themselves, I usually get an answer such as, "Sure, if only it were that easy." My response is always, "Why isn't it that easy?" Why do we feel like the longer we punish ourselves, or the harder we are on ourselves, the more change we will create with this type of negativity? How many times do we need to prove that this doesn't work before we try something new?

Being gentle on yourself is not the same as letting yourself get away with everything. Life creates natural consequences to our actions. It is our natural teacher. There's no need to fear it; just accept that life is going to teach us lessons that will make us stronger, wiser, and more able to experience fulfillment on every level. I want to give you permanent permission to be much easier on yourself! When you feel the mind going toward self-judgment, take a deep breath and repeat after me: "I forgive myself for being perfectly imperfect. I will learn from this and move forward with a stronger mind and a softer heart. Thank you, Universe, for this important lesson."

Learning to trust the Universe creates a tremendous sense of support and relief. This allows us to look at our weight as a lesson, a blessing in disguise. Not every life event unfolds its meaning to us when we first experience it. We must surrender to what is, and trust that at some point we will understand why everything unfolds exactly as it is meant to. It is only now that I understand why I grew up with so much anxiety, and why my weight was the messenger that carried my most important life lessons. This serves as a reminder to me that the real work unfolds itself in the moment we are experiencing it, not after the lesson has presented itself.

There are no food mistakes, no unwanted pounds, and no failed diets that aren't here to teach us something greater about ourselves. These alleged failures hold the key to your food freedom. They are leading you toward the right path. You have to look at them as your guide. They are here to wake you up. What are they telling you?

I believe they tell us to slow down, to put ourselves first, to get clear on what we want. They tell us to let go of the past, embrace the unknown, to write our own story. They teach us that in order to receive all that we want, we have to stop settling for less. We have to do the work. As we deepen our relationship to these important teachers, the work gets easier. We become empowered. Life gets richer. Our bodies begin to change.

From this perspective, there is no right and wrong path or good and bad behavior. What comes up is simply what is, here to show us where we are, in contrast to where we want to be.

Skimmer's Delight

✓ When you put your trust in the Universe, you can relax into your true self.

✓ Who you really are at the core is someone who is full of light, love, trust, forgiveness, and freedom.

✓ When life gets easier, so does healthy eating. Happy people are healthy people.

✓ Forgiveness allows us to learn and move forward with clarity.

✓ Balance is the key to sustainable weight loss.

✓ Your spiritual path is the key to long-lasting happiness.

✓ Your body is a walking reflection of the inner work and fulfillment you create.

Make It Stick

1. Go back through the book and reread the Skimmer's Delights. Make sure you answered all the journal questions in the Make It Stick sections!

2. Set your next health or weight-loss goal, and journal about the logistics of how, with what, and why you are going to get there.
3. Journal about your five biggest takeaways from this book.

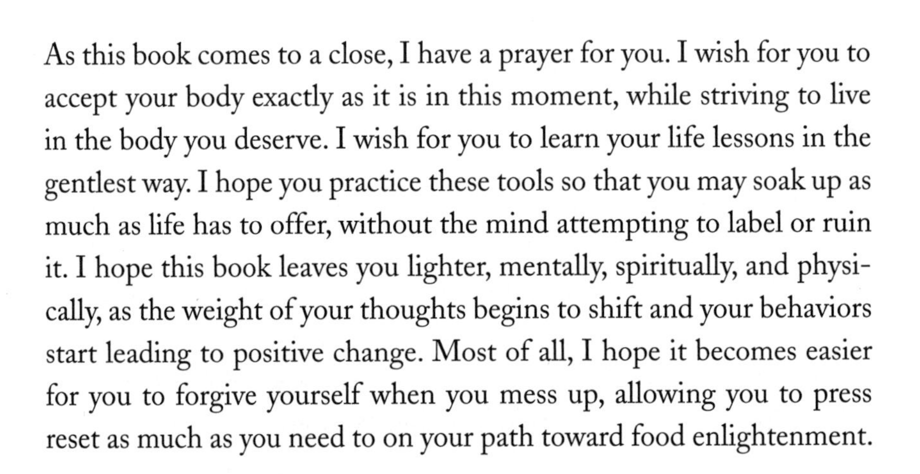

As this book comes to a close, I have a prayer for you. I wish for you to accept your body exactly as it is in this moment, while striving to live in the body you deserve. I wish for you to learn your life lessons in the gentlest way. I hope you practice these tools so that you may soak up as much as life has to offer, without the mind attempting to label or ruin it. I hope this book leaves you lighter, mentally, spiritually, and physically, as the weight of your thoughts begins to shift and your behaviors start leading to positive change. Most of all, I hope it becomes easier for you to forgive yourself when you mess up, allowing you to press reset as much as you need to on your path toward food enlightenment.

appendix

FOODS TO INCLUDE, FOODS TO AVOID, NIBBLES AND SWEET TREATS

FOODS TO INCLUDE

* Superfoods (nutrient-rich foods considered beneficial to health and well-being)

Meat, Poultry, and Fish (Grass-Fed/Pasture-raised/Wild-Caught)

Bacon
Beef
Bone broth
Chicken
Eggs
Fish (salmon, halibut, cod, sea bass)
Lamb
Turkey

Beans and Legumes

Black beans
Cannellini
Edamame (non-GMO)
Garbanzos (chickpeas)
Kidney beans
Lentils
Lima beans
Navy beans
Pinto beans
Split peas

FOODS TO INCLUDE (*continued*)

Grains (Gluten-Free)

Amaranth*
Buckwheat
Millet
Oats
Quinoa*
Rice (brown, red, black, wild)
Sorghum
Teff

Nuts and Seeds

Almonds
Brazil nuts
Chia seeds*
Flaxseed* (freshly ground)
Hempseed*
Macadamia nuts
Pecans
Pine nuts
Pistachios
Pumpkin seeds
Sesame seeds
Sunflower seeds
Walnuts*

Roots

Ginger*
Turmeric*

Starchy "Energy" Vegetables

Beets
Carrots
Jicama
Parsnips
Potatoes (white, yellow, purple, red)
Sweet potatoes / yams
Winter squash (butternut, acorn, pumpkin, etc.)

Nonstarchy Vegetables

Artichokes
Arugula
Asparagus
Bok choy
Broccoli*
Broccolini
Brussels sprouts
Cabbage
Cauliflower
Celery
Chard
Chlorella*
Collard greens
Cucumbers
Dandelion greens
Eggplant
Garlic
Green beans
Kale*
Leeks
Lettuce (except iceberg)
Mushrooms (reishi*, shiitake, portobello, etc.)
Mustard greens
Nori
Okra
Onions
Peppers
Radishes
Scallions/chives
Snap peas
Snow peas
Spinach
Spirulina*
Sprouts*
Summer squash (spaghetti, zucchini, yellow, etc.)
Tomatoes
Wakame
Watercress

Oils and Fats

Avocado oil
Avocados
Butter (grass-fed, such as Kerrygold brand)
Coconut milk (unsweetened)
Coconut oil
Extra-virgin olive oil
Ghee (clarified butter)
MCT oil*
Olives
Sesame oil
Sunflower oil
Walnut oil

Fermented Foods

Coconut yogurt
Kefir
Kimchi*
Miso (organic, non-GMO)
Sauerkraut
Tempeh (organic, non-GMO)

FOODS TO INCLUDE (*continued*)

Fruits

Acai berries*
Apples
Apricots
Bananas
Blackberries
Blueberries
Cherries
Coconuts
Figs
Goji berries*
Grapefruit
Grapes
Kiwi
Lemons
Limes
Mangoes
Oranges
Peaches
Pears
Pineapples
Plums
Pomegranates
Raspberries
Strawberries
Tangerines
Watermelon

Herbs and Spices

Basil
Cayenne
Cilantro
Cinnamon*
Cumin
Dill
Garlic
Ginger*
Mint
Oregano*
Parsley
Rosemary
Turmeric*

Beverages

Bragg Organic Apple Cider Vinegar Drink (unsweetened)
Carbonated water
Flavored water with mint, lemon, basil, ginger, fruit
Four Sigmatic mushroom tea
Golden milk (Gaia Herbs blend)
Herbal tea (Tulsi* is great)
KeVita Sparkling Probiotic Drink
Water*

Sweeteners

Coconut sugar
Dates
Honey
Maple syrup
Stevia (Sweet Leaf brand)

Condiments

Coconut aminos
Hot sauce (Sriracha, Cholula, Yellowbird, etc. — choose ones without preservatives)
Ketchup (organic)
Mayo (avocado or sunflower oil, such as Sir Kensington's brand)
Mustards
Pickles and capers
Salsa (fresh)
Tamari (wheat-free soy sauce)
Tessemae's brand dressings
Vinegar (apple cider*, white/red wine, rice wine, balsamic, etc.)
Worcestershire sauce

FOODS TO AVOID

Artificial Ingredients and Poor-Quality Fats and Oils

- Artificial colors
- Artificial flavors
- Canola oil
- Corn oil
- Fake dairy creamers
- Fat substitutes (margarine, Earth/Smart Balance)
- Food additives
- Food preservatives
- Fried foods
- Oil in plastic containers (always pick colored glass containers!)
- Palm oil
- PAM spray
- Processed meats (deli meats from health food stores are okay)
- Soybean oil
- Trans fats (hydrogenated fats, monoglycerides, diglycerides)
- Vegetable oil

Sugar and White or Refined Carbs

- Artificial sweeteners / sugar substitutes (Splenda, Equal, Sweet'N Low)
- Bread (gluten-free is okay in moderation)
- Chips
- Crackers
- Dried fruits (use as a condiment or sprinkle, not a snack)
- Fruit juice
- High-fructose corn syrup (HFCS) — read every label!
- Iced tea (sweetened)
- Pasta
- Soda/Gatorade
- Tortillas (corn or wheat)

Gluten

Barley
Corn (though gluten-free, it's a reactive grain)
Rye
Seitan
Wheat

Dairy

Cheese (cow, sheep, goat)
Cottage cheese
Cream cheese
Cream/half-and-half
Ice cream
Milk (cow, sheep, goat)
Sour cream
Yogurt (cow, sheep, goat)

Soy

Fake meat (Boca, MorningStar Farms, etc.)
Soybean oil
Tofu

Alcohol

Beer
Liquor
Wine

NIBBLES AND SWEET TREATS

* Recipes found on nutritionalwisdom.com/recipes

Snack Ideas

Almond butter and a half banana
Applegate Farms pepperoni, olives, and Flackers
Apple with pumpkin seeds
Avocado (one half) with sea salt
Avocado cashew dip* with veggies
Avocado egg salad* with raw veggie sticks
Bone broth (pasture-raised, organic)
Chicken salad with grapes and walnuts*
Cucumber and hummus boats*
Egg muffins*
Eggplant roll-ups*
EPIC bars (Bison Bacon Cranberry recommended)
Fruit and a handful of nuts
Green juice (5 g sugar, max)
Guacamole and hummus with sprouts on two slices of roasted eggplant
Hummus deviled eggs*
KIND bars (5 g sugar, max)
Kite Hill's almond cheese
Lemon kale chips*
Nuts / seeds / nut butters (natural)
Oatmega bars (5 g sugar, max)
Olives (handful)
Peanut sauce dip with raw veggies
Precut raw veggies and hummus (think variety: radishes, zucchini, jicama, celery, carrot)
Sea veggies (nori, wakame, hijiki)
Smoked salmon over cucumber with hummus (add dill and capers to be fancy)
Spicy roasted chickpeas*
Turkey breast wrapped with mustard, sprouts, and julienned veggies

Sweet Ideas

- Avocado, carrot, and honey muffins*
- Bragg Organic Apple Cider Vinegar Drink
- Chia pudding* with cinnamon, nuts, fruit, spirulina, chlorella... think smoothie add-ins!
- Coconut yogurt (unsweetened) with hemp, chia, cacao, fruit
- Dates (two) with almond butter
- Easy snack bites*
- "Fudgesicles"— turn your protein shake into popsicles
- Herbal tea with stevia (Yogi, Numi, Tulsi)
- KeVita Sparkling Probiotic Drink
- Lily's chocolate bar (a quarter, max)
- Protein pancakes*
- Raw carrot bites*
- Spicy hot chocolate*

ACKNOWLEDGMENTS

I would like to thank my sister, Mandy Levy, since she was my editor long before I ever wrote a book. She makes sure that the jokes I think are funny are actually funny. She edits my outfits, my writing, my art projects, my home decor, and anything else I can beg her to help me with. Without her I'd be completely uncreative, marginally comical, and very bored a lot of the time. I'd like to thank my husband, Jordan, for putting up with me in general. Everyone who knows us agrees that you deserve a medal. Thank you, Mom, for being the best mom in the world (I can prove this), and for cooking and running my errands for me when I had no time because I had a book deadline. Aaron, thanks for all the brother-sister walks and business talks when I needed to run through my ideas. Thank you to the Nutritional Wisdom team. You are magic, and I am lucky to share my vision with you. My dad didn't really do much for this book, but I have to thank him because without him, everything in my house would stay broken and unhung, and I would not be the razor-sharp businesswoman and expert negotiator that I am today. Last, thank you to baby Tillie, who was growing in my belly while I wrote this book. You kicked me a bunch and gave me massive indigestion while I was writing, but I wrote this book so that when you grow up, you can love your body unconditionally and find lasting health and happiness.

NOTES

Chapter 4. Is Stress Stressing You Out?

Page 50, *"a positive form of stress"*: *Merriam-Webster*, s.v. "eustress," accessed October 15, 2018, https://www.merriam-webster.com/dictionary/eustress.

Page 51, *In her incredible book* The Fear Cure: Lissa Rankin, *The Fear Cure: Cultivating Courage as Medicine for the Body, Mind, and Soul* (Carlsbad, CA: Hay House, 2016), introduction.

Chapter 5. One Size Fits No One

Page 72, *Their book,* The Metabolic Typing Diet: William Wolcott and Trish Fahey, *The Metabolic Typing Diet* (New York: Broadway, 2000).

Page 73, *"Just like a computer"*: David Allen, *Getting Things Done: The Art of Stress-Free Productivity* (New York: Penguin, 2015), 70 (italics mine).

Chapter 6. Conscious Eating

Page 84, *As Eckhart Tolle teaches*: Eckhart Tolle, *The Power of Now: A Guide to Spiritual Enlightenment* (Novato, CA: New World Library, 2004), 12, 226.

Chapter 9. Life Is Best When You Manifest

Page 130, *"All potential experiences"*: Joe Dispenza, *Breaking the Habit of Being Yourself* (Carlsbad, CA: Hay House, 2013), 21.

INDEX

ABOUT THE AUTHOR

Carly Pollack is the founder of Nutritional Wisdom, a thriving holistic health private practice based in Austin, Texas. She is a certified clinical nutritionist specializing in holistic nutrition and spiritual advancement. Carly has been awarded Best Nutritionist in Austin four years running and has helped more than fifteen thousand people achieve their health and happiness goals. Carly has lectured all over the country for incredible organizations such as Facebook, Whole Foods Market, Texas Women's Conference, Livestrong Foundation, Lululemon, Atlassian, Frog Design, WeWork, Techstars, Flatwater Foundation, and the Texas Medical Association, among many more.

To sign up for Carly's weekly newsletters and free advice, go to www.carlypollack.com. For individual coaching, check out her private practice at www.nutritionalwisdom.com.

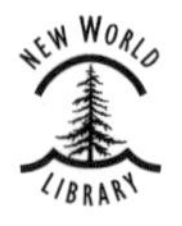

NEW WORLD LIBRARY is dedicated to publishing books and other media that inspire and challenge us to improve the quality of our lives and the world.

We are a socially and environmentally aware company. We recognize that we have an ethical responsibility to our readers, our authors, our staff members, and our planet.

We serve our readers by creating the finest publications possible on personal growth, creativity, spirituality, wellness, and other areas of emerging importance. We serve our authors by working with them to produce and promote quality books that reach a wide audience. We serve New World Library employees with generous benefits, significant profit sharing, and constant encouragement to pursue their most expansive dreams.

Whenever possible, we print our books with soy-based ink on 100 percent postconsumer-waste recycled paper. We power our offices with solar energy and contribute to nonprofit organizations working to make the world a better place for us all.

Our products are available wherever books are sold. Visit our website to download our catalog, subscribe to our e-newsletter, read our blog, and link to authors' websites, videos, and podcasts.

customerservice@newworldlibrary.com
Phone: 415-884-2100 or 800-972-6657
Orders: Ext. 10 • Catalog requests: Ext. 10
Fax: 415-884-2199

www.newworldlibrary.com